Stories for Nurses
英語コラムで読む看護師の物語

 原著 K. Lynn Wieck　 編著 田中 芳文　 著 廣渡 太郎
　山﨑 麻由美
　片岡 由美子

看護の科学新社

看護師をめざす日本のみなさんへ

—原著者からのメッセージ

　私は，自分が経験した看護のストーリーをみなさんと共有できることを，とても嬉しく，そして光栄に思います。私はこれまで，他者を援助したり，学生たちを指導したりしてきましたが，看護の第一線を退いた現在もそのことに感謝する日々です。みなさんはとても崇高な職業を選ばれました。今後のみなさんの看護師としてのキャリアが，私と同じように幸せで満足いくものになることを願っています。最後に，今回このような素晴らしい機会を与えていただいたことに感謝するとともに，みなさんの看護師としての将来が，豊かで実りあるものになることを心から祈ります。

K. Lynn Wieck, RN, PhD

はしがき

　急速に進歩する現代の保健医療の世界では，看護師たちの長所や功績といったものが見落とされ，看護の否定的な面ばかり強調される傾向があります。多忙を極める仕事に追われる看護師たち自身も，看護という仕事の幸福な瞬間や喜びを忘れがちです。しかし，看護が抱える現実の問題を認めると同時に，看護の肯定的な側面にもっと目を向けることによって，看護をよりよいものにする必要があります。米国テキサス大学タイラー校看護保健科学部で長年に看護学生を指導した経験のあるK. Lynn Wieck教授は，そう主張する人物のひとりです。本書は，彼女が米国の有力紙 *Houston Chronicle* に連載した看護に関するコラムから選りすぐった15編を題材に作成した，看護学生のための英語学習用テキストです。

　本書は15のUnitから構成されています。各Unitでは，まず予習としてVocabulary Checkに取り組んでください。英文にはできる限り多くの注を付けて，なるべく辞書を引かなくても読み進めることができるようにしてあります。本文に関係するA（内容理解），B（書き取り），C（英文整序）と，それとは別のD（看護分野の単語）から構成されています。本文と練習問題Bの音源も用意してありますので利用してください。

　本書が，わが国で看護師をめざす学生のこころに響き，その英語学習に少しでも役立つことを願っています。

　最後に，本書出版の意義にご理解をいただいた看護の科学新社に敬意を表しますとともに，出版のためにご尽力くださった同社代表取締役の濱崎浩一さんにこころより感謝申し上げます。

2022年初秋

編著者

編著者（2022年11月末現在）

◉ **田中 芳文**　たなか よしふみ
島根県立大学人間文化学部教授
編集およびUnit 1〜6執筆担当

◉ **廣渡 太郎**　ひろわたり たろう
日本赤十字秋田看護大学教授
Unit 7，10，11執筆担当

◉ **山﨑 麻由美**　やまさき まゆみ
神戸常盤大学保健科学部教授
Unit 8，12，13執筆担当

◉ **片岡 由美子**　かたおか ゆみこ
愛知県立大学看護学部准教授
Unit 9，14，15執筆担当

Contents

表紙デザイン・本文DTP／スタジオ・コア
表紙・本文イラスト／櫻田耕司

本書の使い方

◎**音声教材について**

　本文中の [Audio] マーク箇所（本文・練習問題B）につきましては，朗読音声をご用意しております。小社サイト（https://kangonokagaku.co.jp）上の本書ページからMP3データがダウンロードできます。必要時にお使いください。

Unit 1 The Joy of Nursing

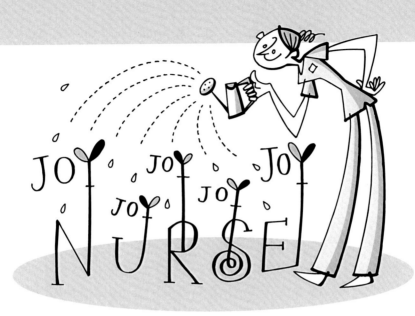

Vocabulary Check

次の日本語に相当する英語を下から選んで記入しなさい。

1 (   )　心配，懸念
2 (   )　否定主義，消極主義
3 (   )　悲しみ
4 (   )　患者
5 (   )　同僚
6 (   )　道具，装置
7 (   )　会計士
8 (   )　出来事
9 (   )　特権
10 (   )　明るさ，輝き

accountant ／ brightness ／ concern ／ gadget ／ incident ／ negativism ／
patient ／ peer ／ privilege ／ sorrow

1　　I love being a nurse! I'm not ashamed to say it. Nursing brings me joy every day of my life.

　　However, one of the concerns I have for both the current and the future workforce in nursing is the rampant amount of negativism. It
5 seems that not enough positive things are being said about the nursing profession these days.

　　When you read about nursing in most newspapers and in magazines, the focus is mainly on how managed care is ruining everything. The healthcare picture portrayed in public media is usually very negative.

10　　So, who is talking about the joys of being a nurse? If everything we read depicts the sorrows and horrors of nursing, can we expect to attract bright and dedicated young people into our profession?

　　It is past time for someone to talk about the joy of nursing.

　　True, there are a lot of days when nurses probably live closer to the
15 negatives of managed care than the joys of being a nurse. When you are tired, overworked, underappreciated, and fearful for your license, it can be difficult to remember why you became a nurse in the first place.

　　Let's begin by talking about that "feeling." You know the one I am talking about?

Notes

1	be ashamed to ～／～するのが恥ずかしい	*11*	depict／描く
3	both A and B／A も B も	*11*	horror／恐怖
3	current／現在の	*12*	dedicated／ひたむきな，献身的な
4	workforce／労働力人口	*14*	the negatives／問題点，欠点
4	rampant／すさまじい，途方もない	*16*	underappreciated／正しく評価されていない
4	It seems that ～／～のようだ，～らしい	*16*	fearful／心配して，不安で
8	managed care／管理医療	*17*	in the first place／そもそも
8	ruin／だめにする，台なしにする	*18*	begin by ～ing／～することからはじめる

1 It's that feeling you get when you reach deep inside your professional nurse self and do something that lights up the whole room. Maybe you are the only one who sees it. Maybe a patient, family, or peer sees it. Maybe the whole unit sees it. The important thing, however, is that **you**
5 see it. You know when you do well, when you make a difference.

You also must know that sweet feeling deep in your inner self that flashes like electricity into your fingertips and your toes and makes you feel lighter than air. It's that feeling that spreads to your brain where a slight smile cannot be repressed, and you fear your whole head must be
10 glowing like a neon sign in the darkness.

Then you look back at what you did, and you know you made a difference. You know it was extraordinary, and you savor the moment with this thought: "This is why I wanted to become a nurse!"

I think nurses are blessed with this feeling, although I imagine
15 engineers get it, too, when their gadgets actually work. Maybe accountants get it when column A actually equals column B. I imagine teachers get it when a student finally grasps a concept or figures out a problem. But in nursing, we are so fortunate that incidents which trigger the feeling come often and leave us feeling invincible.

Notes

2	light up ～／～を明るくする	13	This is why ～／こういうわけで～
4	unit／病棟，部門	14	be blessed with ～／～に恵まれている
5	do well／成功する，うまくやる		
5	make a difference／重要である，影響を与える	16	column／(縦の)欄
		16	equal／等しい
7	fingertip／指先	17	grasp／理解する，把握する
8	it's A that ～／～するのはAである	17	concept／概念，考え
8	spread／広がる	17	figure out ～／～を解く
8	brain／脳	18	so ～ that...／とても～なので…
9	repress／抑える，こらえる	18	fortunate／恵まれている，幸せな
11	look back at ～／～を振り返る	19	trigger／起こす，招く
12	extraordinary／並外れた，驚くべき	19	invincible／揺るぎない，不屈の
12	savor／かみしめる，堪能する		

1   Remember when that patient crashed? You looked at the situation and knew just what to do with precision and compassion. Maybe a student or two were watching in awe and admiration. Your actions made a difference in a person's life. What an awesome privilege!

5   This special feeling is the essence of the joy of nursing.

   I had one of those feelings recently when a perfect stranger came up to me and said, "You don't know me. I'm a nurse. I hated my job and had decided to get out of nursing recently, but I read your column [titled] 'My Most Unforgettable Patient,' and I remembered why I

10 became a nurse. I decided I could never give that up, so I changed jobs, and I'm so much happier."

   I thanked her for her kind words and continued along my path, as did she. But I kept wondering whether people were noticing the sudden brightness from my glowing head, or if they wondered what I was

15 smiling about. It's that "feeling" ! It's why I became a nurse.

Notes

1	crash／心拍停止状態になる	*8*	column／特別寄稿欄，コラム
2	with precision and compassion／正確に，そして思いやりをもって	*10*	give ～ up／～をやめる，～を捨てる
3	in awe and admiration／畏敬と賞賛のまなざしで	*12*	thank A for B／AにBを感謝する
4	awesome／すばらしい	*13*	keep ～ing／～してばかりいる
6	come up to ～／～に近寄る	*13*	wonder whether ～／～かしらと思う
8	get out of ～／～から逃げ出す	*13*	wonder if ～／～かしらと思う

練習問題

A 次の英文が，本文の内容と一致する場合にはＴを，一致しない場合にはＦを（　　）内に記入しなさい。

（　　）1 I love being a nurse, but I'm ashamed to say it.

（　　）2 Negative things are often said about the nursing profession these days.

（　　）3 There are many days when nurses live closer to the joys of being a nurse than the negatives of managed care.

（　　）4 Nurses and teachers get that special "feeling," but engineers and accountants do not.

（　　）5 A certain nurse read my column and remembered why she became a nurse.

B 音声を聴いて，英文の（　　）内に適語を記入しなさい。

1 Why do you want to become a nurse （　　　　　　）（　　　　　　）

（　　　　　　）（　　　　　　）？

2 She （　　　　　　）（　　　　　　）（　　　　　　） why she had come.

3 The nurse spoke （　　　　　　）（　　　　　　）.

4 I wanted to （　　　　　　）（　　　　　　）（　　　　　　） the group.

5 We would like to （　　　　　　） everyone （　　　　　　） helping.

C 日本文に合うように，（　）内の語句を並べかえて英文を作りなさい。

1 私たちに選択の余地はないようだ。
(that, it, choice, we, seems, no, have).

_____

2 こういうわけで私たちはその公園に行くことを断る。
(why, to, is, this, to, refuse, the park, we, go).

_____

3 とても寒かったので，ジャネットは震えていた。
(was, Janet, so, shivering, it, that, cold, was).

_____

D 次の英語に相当する日本語を下から選び，記号で答えなさい【呼吸器系，循環器系，免疫系，内分泌系】。

1 throat（　　）2 larynx（　　）3 trachea（　　）4 bronchus（　　）

5 lung（　　）6 heart（　　）7 coronary artery（　　）

8 bone marrow（　　）9 spleen（　　）10 thyroid gland（　　）

ア．骨髄	イ．喉頭	ウ．気管支	エ．心臓	オ．気管
カ．脾臓	キ．冠状動脈	ク．咽喉	ケ．肺	コ．甲状腺

Unit 2

Milestones

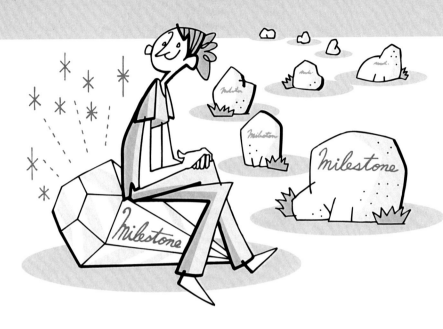

Vocabulary Check

次の日本語に相当する英語を下から選んで記入しなさい。

1. (   ) 講堂
2. (   ) 離婚
3. (   ) 満足
4. (   ) 安心，安堵
5. (   ) 失望，落胆
6. (   ) 存在
7. (   ) 治療
8. (   ) 苦しみ，苦痛
9. (   ) 大混乱
10. (   ) 大成功

auditorium ／ chaos ／ dismay ／ divorce ／ healing ／ presence ／ relief ／
satisfaction ／ suffering ／ triumph

Audio 1

Recently, my husband and I proudly watched as our third (and last) son graduated from college. As we sat in the huge auditorium packed with families and friends, I was struck by the significance of these types of events in people's lives.

5 Think back over the milestones in your life. A milestone is a significant event in a person's life history. I wonder how many of these milestones relate to your chosen profession.

When we think of significant events, we usually think of things like births and weddings. Completion of an educational program and 10 receiving awards are also significant. Some milestones are not so positive, such as deaths and divorces, but we remember and celebrate our capacity to overcome sadness and to go on with our lives.

What are the hallmarks of a milestone? We usually take a lot of photos and have friends and family around us. An emotional response is 15 involved, and the event is remembered and recalled, often for years to come. The best part is a feeling of accomplishment and satisfaction. In healthcare, however, our milestones are often more subtle.

Think about the milestones in your professional career. One would certainly be the completion of your education. Your graduation or

Notes

	milestone／重要な出来事	9	completion／修了
2	(be) packed with ～／～で込み合っている	10	award／賞
		11	such as ～／たとえば～のような
3	be struck by ～／～で感銘を受ける	11	celebrate／ほめたたえる
3	significance／重要性	12	overcome／乗り越える
5	think back over ～／～のことを振り返る，思い出す	12	go on with ～／～を続ける
		13	hallmark／特徴，特質
6	significant／重要な	15	involve／伴う
6	I wonder ～／～かしらと思う	15	A to come／これから先のA
7	relate to ～／～と関係がある	16	accomplishment／達成，成就
7	chosen／(好きで)選んだ	17	healthcare／保健医療
8	think of ～／～を思い出す	17	subtle／微妙な，目立たない

1   pinning held a special moment of accomplishment and pride for you and your family.

    Remember the feelings of relief and excitement as you entered your chosen career. Remember your uncertainty about being able to do the
5   job well. How about your confidence that you could go out and fix all the problems that were plaguing healthcare—and your dismay at finding out what the real world was like? That milestone still brings back a lot of mixed emotions for me.

    Do you remember your first real accomplishment as a new healthcare
10 professional? Maybe it was the first IV you started on a patient with impossible veins, the first time you had the instrument in the physician's hands before the word was even spoken, the family who came back to tell you how much your words and presence meant to them in a crisis.

    During my first six months as a nurse on a urology unit, we had an
15 overflow plastic surgery patient. The plastic surgeon, unhappy at having to visit a urology floor in the first place, stopped in the middle of a dressing change and complimented me on how well I had cut the gauze so it would not ravel and interfere with the healing of his tiny, precise stitches. For heaven's sake, he complimented me on cutting a straight

Notes

1	pinning／（看護教育プログラム卒業を表す）ピン付きの記章 (pin) を受け取ること
4	uncertainty／不確かさ
5	How about ～?／～についてはどうか?
5	confidence／自信，確信
5	go out and ～／努力して何とか～する
5	fix／解決する
6	plague／苦しめる，悩ます
7	find out／知る，発見する
7	bring back ～／～を思い返させる
8	mixed／入り交じった
10	IV／静脈注射，点滴 (intravenous)
10	patient／患者
11	vein／静脈 (cf. artery「動脈」)
11	instrument／器具，器械
11	physician／医師
13	crisis／危機，(病気が回復するかどうかの)峠
14	urology unit／泌尿器科病棟
15	overflow／あふれ出た
15	plastic surgery／形成外科
15	plastic surgeon／形成外科医
16	in the first place／そもそも
16	in the middle of ～／～の最中に
17	dressing change／包帯交換
17	compliment A on ～／～についてAをほめる
17	gauze／ガーゼ
18	so (that) A will not ～／Aが～しないように
18	ravel／もつれる
18	interfere with ～／～のじゃまをする，～を妨げる
18	tiny／ごく小さな
18	precise／正確な
19	stitch／(縫合する際の)一針
19	for heaven's sake／(驚きを表して)なんとまあ

line, but I felt like I had been awarded the Medal of Honor and still remember his words these 32 years later.

I had put the patient's needs ahead of my own busy schedule, and someone had noticed. What a great feeling!

What about your first patient death? That is a milestone for many of us. Do you realize how privileged we are to assist at people's deaths? Remember that first time one of your patients died, and the family looked to you for comfort and guidance? That was the time that you found out that you did, indeed, know what to say and whom to call. You could see the relief in the family's eyes that someone had control in a situation that they could not control. It was one of those wonderful, precious moments in nursing when you know you are needed and your actions ease the pain and suffering of another person.

Unfortunately, in the hectic chaos of healthcare today, it seems that the acknowledgment of milestones has gotten lost. We are so busy just trying to cope with the complex world that we do not have time to celebrate special moments. It is like treading water. We aren't sinking, but we aren't making a lot of progress either.

I strongly urge you to recognize the new discoveries in your own

---

Notes

1	feel like ～／～のような気がする	14	unfortunately／不幸にも
1	award／授与する	14	hectic／てんてこ舞いの
1	the Medal of Honor／(米国の軍人に対する)名誉勲章	14	it seems that ～／～のようだ，～らしい
3	ahead of ～／～より先に	15	acknowledgement／認めること
5	What about ～?／～についてはどうか？	15	so ～that...／とても～なので…
6	privileged to ～／～して光栄な	15	busy ～ing／～するのに忙しい
8	look to A for B／AにBを期待する	16	cope with ～／～に対処する
8	comfort／慰め	17	tread water／立ち泳ぎをする
9	indeed／本当に，確かに	18	make progress／前進する
12	precious／貴重な，大切な	19	urge A to ～／Aに～するようしきりに勧める

1 practice. Pat yourself on the back when you take a big step, or even a small one. Promotions, recognition, triumphs—we should all celebrate them because they are part of the special commitment we have made to serve the health needs of the public.

Notes

1 pat A on the back／Aをよくやった とほめる

1 take a big step／大きな一歩を踏み 出す

2 promotion／昇進

2 recognition／表彰

3 make a commitment to ～／～する と誓う，～すると約束する

4 serve／役に立つ

練習問題

A 本文の内容に合うように，次の英文の（　　）内に入る語を下から選びなさい。

1 A milestone is a significant event in a person's life（　　　　　）.

2 The best part of a milestone is a（　　　　　）of accomplishment and satisfaction.

3 The plastic surgeon complimented me in the middle of dressing （　　　　　）.

4 Your first patient（　　　　　）is a milestone for many of us.

5 Unfortunately, we do not have（　　　　　）to celebrate milestones.

death／time／change／feeling／history

B 音声を聴いて，次の英文の（　　）内に適切な語を記入しなさい。

1 Fatty foods（　　　　　）（　　　　　）French fries are not good for you.

2 （　　　　　）（　　　　　）that hurricane last night?

3 He（　　　　　）the six-year-old girl（　　　　　）her good manners.

4 I always arrived（　　　　　）（　　　　　）the others.

5 The patient（　　　　　）（　　　　　）the pain of cancer and finally got well again.

C 次の日本文に合うように，（　　）内の語句を並べかえて英文を作りなさい。

① 今日は雨になるだろうか。
(it, today, wonder, will, whether, I, rain).

_____

② 電話がかかってきたときは夕食の最中だった。
(in, of, rang, the middle, when, we, the phone, were, dinner).

_____

③ メアリーは雪の中で寒くないように暖かい服を着ていた。
(she, so, cold, warm clothes, the snow, wore, wouldn't, Mary, be, in).

_____

D 次の英語に相当する日本語を下から選び，記号で答えなさい【消化器系，泌尿器系，生殖器系】。

① esophagus（　　）② stomach（　　）③ liver（　　）

④ pancreas（　　）⑤ small intestine（　　）⑥ rectum（　　）

⑦ colon（　　）⑧ kidney（　　）⑨ bladder（　　）⑩ uterus（　　）

ア．腎臓　イ．直腸　ウ．胃　エ．膀胱　オ．食道
カ．子宮　キ．膵臓　ク．小腸　ケ．肝臓　コ．結腸

Unit 3

My Most Unforgettable Patient

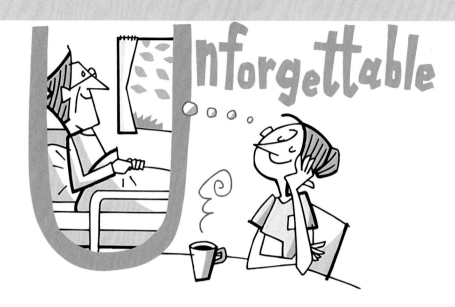

Vocabulary Check

次の日本語に相当する英語を下から選んで記入しなさい。

① (	)	ためらい，躊躇
② (	)	同僚
③ (	)	依頼人，顧客
④ (	)	金銭出納係，窓口係
⑤ (	)	治療，処置
⑥ (	)	激励
⑦ (	)	無力，どうしようもないこと
⑧ (	)	深い理解，見識
⑨ (	)	見物人，傍観者
⑩ (	)	投入，傾注

client／colleague／encouragement／helplessness／hesitation／insight／
investment／spectator／teller／treatment

Audio

1   Every nurse has had that special patient who will be remembered forever. Regardless of the passage of time or the circumstances of the encounter, all nurses can tell you about their most unforgettable patients without any hesitation.

5   To reassure myself of this point, I posed this question to a colleague: "If I asked you about your most unforgettable patient, could you tell me?" In less than a second she responded, "Of course. I had just finished my shift in CCU, and she took my hand and begged me not to leave so she would not have to die alone. She had no family, so I stayed
10 at her bedside all night until she died, just before daybreak. She never let go of my hand."

   Your most unforgettable patient may bring up happy memories or sad ones, but one of the best things about being a nurse is the times you get to share with patients.

15   What other profession can boast about having the privilege of sharing the most intimate, the most critical, the most life-altering moments of their clients' lives? Do you ever hear accountants talk about their most unforgettable ledger sheets or bank tellers talk about their most unforgettable bank accounts? Probably not.

Notes

unforgettable／忘れられない，記憶に残る
1 patient／患者
2 regardless of 〜／〜に関係なく
2 passage／経過
2 circumstance／事情，状況
3 encounter／出会い
5 reassure／安心させる
5 pose／提起する，持ち出す
7 less than 〜／〜より少ない
8 shift／(交代制の)勤務時間
8 CCU／冠状動脈疾患集中治療室 (coronary care unit) (心疾患集中治療室 (cardiac care unit)，心血管疾患集中治療室 (cardiovascular care unit)，重傷治療室(critical care unit) を表す場合もある)
8 beg A not to 〜／Aに〜しないよう懇願する
9 so (that) A will not 〜／Aが〜しないように
10 daybreak／夜明け
11 let go of 〜／〜を離す
12 bring up 〜／〜を持ち出す
14 get to 〜／〜するようになる
14 share A with B／AをBと共有する
15 boast about 〜／〜を自慢する
15 privilege／特権
16 intimate／個人的な，私的な
16 critical／重大な，危機の
16 life-altering／人生を変えてしまうような
17 accountant／会計士
18 ledger／元帳，出納簿
19 account／口座

1　In healthcare, we are there when human beings experience those dynamic moments that make them human. We are there during birth, at the time of death, during pain and the relief of pain. We share life-altering decisions and body-altering treatments. We offer support,
5　encouragement, and friendship. What a precious gift—to be able to share these most intimate and important times of our patients' lives.

　But sharing critical moments means we also share the happiness, sadness, fear, frustration, anger, and helplessness of these emotional times. We see patients at their best and at their worst. And it is through
10　these privileged insights that we can remember those unforgettable patients. It is also an important part of what makes our lives and our careers so interesting and so enjoyable.

　I am not going to tell you about my most unforgettable patient. Instead, I would invite you to take a moment or two to remember your
15　most unforgettable patient. Remember the emotions surrounding the encounter. Whether the experience was happy or sad, funny or embarrassing, gratifying or frightening, remember that every day a part of your professional life is spent making a difference in people's lives.

　As you search your memory for those significant moments in your

Notes

2	dynamic／絶えず変化する		〜する
3	relief／除去，軽減	*15*	surround／取り巻く，包む
4	body-altering／身体を変えてしまうような	*16*	whether A or B／AであろうとBであろうと
5	precious／貴重な，大切な	*17*	embarrassing／恥ずかしい，気まずい
5	be able to 〜／〜できる		
9	at one's best／最高の状態で	*17*	gratifying／満足を与える，愉快な
9	at one's worst／最悪の状態で	*17*	frightening／恐ろしい，ぎょっとさせるような
9	it is A that 〜／〜なのはAである．		
10	privileged／特権を与えられた	*18*	make a difference／重要である，影響を与える
14	instead／その代わりに		
14	invite A to 〜／Aに〜するよう勧める	*19*	search A for B／Bを求めてAを捜す
14	take a moment to 〜／時間を取って	*19*	significant／重要な

1 nursing career, rejoice that you have chosen a career that is built on being involved in the lives of others. Many people in this world go to work every day uninspired and unmotivated. They have jobs that earn them a living, but really don't make that much difference. They

5 contribute their time, but they hold back their selves. They show up each day, but they never get involved. One of the joys of nursing is that it is not a spectator profession—you have to get involved.

This investment of your whole heart and soul is what makes you a special nurse. It is also what makes your patients special. As you

10 remember that one patient who was most special, remember that he or she benefited from the fact that you decided to be a nurse.

There are many joys in being a nurse. Every day, you share your healing gifts with people who need you so much. I can only hope that one day when one of your patients is asked, "Tell me about your most

15 unforgettable nurse," he or she will smile and, without hesitation, share a happy and healing moment spent with you.

Notes

1	rejoice／喜ぶ	5	show up／姿を現す
2	be involved in 〜／〜に関わりがある	6	get involved／関係する，関与する
3	uninspired and unmotivated／平凡にこれといった動機もなく	8	whole heart and soul／全身全霊
		11	benefit／利益を得る
3	earn A B／AにBをもたらす	11	the fact that 〜／〜という事実
4	living／生計，生活費	13	healing／癒すような
5	contribute／捧げる，与える	14	one day／いつか，ある日
5	hold back／とっておく，抑える	15	share／伝える，話す

練習問題

A 本文の内容に合うように,次の英文の（　　　）内に入る語を下から選びなさい。

① All nurses can tell you about their most unforgettable patients without any （　　　　　）.

② One of the best things about being a nurse is the （　　　　　） you get to share with patients.

③ Other profession can not boast about having （　　　　　） of sharing the most critical moments of their clients' lives.

④ Nurses spend their professional life making a （　　　　　） in people's life.

⑤ One of the joys of nursing is that it is not a （　　　　　） profession.

```
difference/spectator/times/privilege/hesitation
```

B 音声を聴いて，次の英文の（　　　）内に適切な語を記入しなさい。

① The law requires equal treatment for all, （　　　　　）（　　　　　） race, religion, age, or sex.

② There were （　　　　）（　　　　） five nurses in the nurses' station.

③ A monkey （　　　　）（　　　　）（　　　　） a branch and dropped to the ground.

④ He was （　　　）（　　　）（　　　　） in the freestyle competition.

⑤ She （　　　　）（　　　　） late for the meeting.

C 次の日本文に合うように，（　　）内の語句を並べかえて英文を作りなさい。

① 私は彼にそんなに速く車を運転しないように懇願した。
（fast, him, drive, to, begged, not, I, so）.

② 彼らがドイツへ行ったのは去年だった。
（that, Germany, last year, went, was, to, they, it）.

③ 私は彼が死んだという事実を受け入れることができない。
（dead, is, that, I, the fact, accept, he, cannot）.

D 次の英語に相当する日本語を下から選び，記号で答えなさい【症状や徴候①】。

① cough（　　） ② sore throat（　　） ③ nausea（　　）

④ diarrhea（　　） ⑤ constipation（　　） ⑥ dizziness（　　）

⑦ convulsion（　　） ⑧ obesity（　　） ⑨ dehydration（　　）

⑩ itching（　　）

> ア．けいれん　イ．吐き気　ウ．かゆみ　エ．脱水　オ．咳
> カ．めまい　キ．便秘　ク．喉の痛み　ケ．下痢　コ．肥満

Unit 4
Humor is Good for What Ails You!

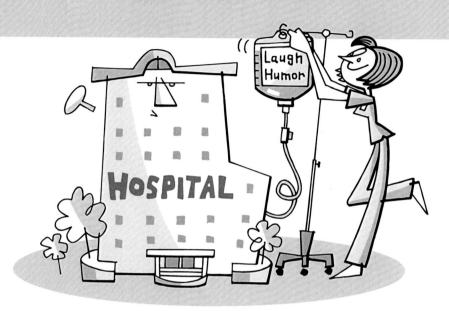

Vocabulary Check

次の日本語に相当する英語を下から選んで記入しなさい。

1 (　　　　　　　) （血液の）循環，血行
2 (　　　　　　　) 呼吸
3 (　　　　　　　) 器具，設備
4 (　　　　　　　) 動機，目的
5 (　　　　　　　) 服用量
6 (　　　　　　　) 挫傷，打撲傷
7 (　　　　　　　) 出血
8 (　　　　　　　) 包帯
9 (　　　　　　　) 薬，薬剤
10 (　　　　　　　) 同僚

bandage／bleeding／bruise／circulation／coworker／dose／equipment／medication／motive／respiration

1   We've all heard it, but is laughter really the best medicine? Research has shown that one good, deep belly laugh per day is good for circulation, respiration, agitation, and probably constipation.

So if laughter is so good for us, why is it so rare?

5   Healthcare has been a great beneficiary of technological advancements. Many lives are saved each year because of the modern equipment, medicines, and techniques available.

So why aren't we happier about it? It appears to me that the mood in hospitals has grown increasingly somber.

10   Although I recognize that a hospital is not a comedy club, I believe the absence of laughter is not therapeutic or even healthy. What has happened? Where did all the laughter go?

I would like to propose a possible answer. Hospitals have always been serious business. People die there. Lives are changed forever in

15   hospitals, and that has always been the case.

I invite you to walk down the halls of a hospital and count the number of people you see smiling or laughing. Nurses used to spread sunshine and cheer along with medicines and back rubs. I propose that the cheer has gone the same route as the back rubs. No one has time

---

Notes

	ail／苦しめる，悩ます	11	absence／欠如
1	medicine／薬	11	therapeutic／治療に役立つ
2	good／十分な，かなりの	13	would like to ～／～したい
2	deep／心の底からの	13	propose／提案する
2	belly／腹	15	be the case／事実である，実情である
2	per day／1日につき	16	invite A to ～／Aに～するよう勧める
3	agitation／興奮，不安	16	the number of ～／～の数
3	constipation／便秘	17	used to ～／かつては～したものだ
5	healthcare／保健医療	17	spread／広める
5	beneficiary／受益者	18	along with ～／～に加えて，～といっしょに
6	advancement／進歩，向上		
6	because of ～／～が原因で，～のために	18	back／背中
		18	rub／マッサージ
7	available／利用できる，入手可能な	19	have gone／存在しない，なくなる
8	it appears (to A) that ～／(Aには)～と思われる	19	the same A as B／Bと同じ(ような)A
9	somber／陰気な，憂鬱な	19	no one ～ anymore／もはや誰も～でない

■21

1   anymore.

    "Oh, great," you are probably moaning,

    "One more thing for me to do—be a little ray of sunshine."

    I know that your patients would benefit from an occasional smile, but
5 my motives are not that pure. I am being terribly selfish. I think that a
happy nurse is a healthy and more competent nurse.

    Who do you want to administer your Coumadin dose—the nurse who
is smiling and chatting with you about the small bruise on your ankle
that has not gotten any bigger, or the nurse who is frowning while
10 trying to remember all of the things to be done before shift change and
who ignores the new bleeding on your bandage? Your choice.

    I firmly believe we take ourselves too seriously in this world,
especially in nursing. Try to differentiate between those times when
seriousness is essential and when it is an unnecessary encumbrance.

15   While you are figuring out my medication dose or determining my IV
rate, I want "serious." But when you are trying to decide who goes to
lunch first or who will work the double shift to cover for a colleague
who is ill, a little humor can be a wonderful ally.

    Sick patients need to see a smile. They need to hear a laugh. Even if

Notes

2 moan／うめき声を出す	*12* take oneself seriously／真剣に考える
3 ray／光, 輝き	
4 patient／患者	*13* differentiate between A and B／AとBを区別する
4 benefit／利益を得る	
4 occasional／時折の	*14* seriousness／真剣さ
5 selfish／自己中心的な	*14* encumbrance／邪魔物
6 competent／有能な	*15* figure out／計算する
7 administer／(薬を)投与する	*15* IV／点滴 (intravenous)
7 Coumadin／クーマディン(抗凝血薬)	*16* rate／速度
8 chat／雑談する	*17* double shift／連続勤務
8 ankle／足首	*17* cover for 〜／〜の代わりをする
9 frown／顔をしかめる	*17* colleague／同僚
10 shift／(交代制の)勤務時間	*18* ally／味方, 協力者
11 ignore／無視する	*19* even if 〜／たとえ〜だとしても
12 firmly／断固として	

1   they cannot laugh themselves because of tubes or pain, they need the hope that laughter is not far away. Sometimes hope is all we can offer people. I believe that laughter and happiness are things worth hoping and waiting for.

5   So I urge all of you to have at least one good laugh per day. If you are really desperate, buy a humor book or an issue of *Reader's Digest*. Look at the humor in situations.

   A glass is either half empty or half full—it just depends on how you look at it. Step back and make yourself take a deep breath before you

10   snap at someone. Laugh at the absurdity of the situation and go forward. You will not only be a much sought-after ally by your coworkers, but you will also like yourself better, too.

   Brighten up your world with some laughter and some cheer. Don't worry that you might miss some of the problems in healthcare; there

15   will always be plenty of people anxious to point out what's wrong. What we need in nursing is more people pointing out what's right. It is wonderful to be a nurse. Enjoy yourself!

Notes

2	far away／遠くに
3	worth ～ing／～する価値がある
5	urge A to ～／Aに～するようしきりに勧める
5	at least／少なくとも
6	desperate／絶望した，自暴自棄の
6	issue／（雑誌・新聞などの）～号
6	*Reader's Digest*／『リーダーズダイジェスト』(米国のポケットサイズの月刊誌，1922創刊)
8	either A or B／AかBかいずれか
8	depend on ～／～による，～次第である
9	step back／一歩引いてみる，距離をおいて考える
9	take a deep breath／深呼吸する
10	snap at ～／～にがみがみ言う
10	absurdity／ばからしさ
10	go forward／前進する
11	not only A but also B／AだけでなくBもまた
11	sought-after／引っ張りだこの
13	brighten up ～／～を明るくする
14	miss／見落とす
15	plenty of ～／たくさんの～
15	anxious to ～／～することを切望して
16	point out ～／～を指摘する

練習問題

A 本文の内容に合うように, 次の英文の ( ) 内に入る語を下から選びなさい。

1 Nurses used to spread (   ) and cheer.

2 Many lives are saved each year because of modern equipment, medicine, and (   ).

3 The mood in (   ) has grown gloomy.

4 If you are really desperate, look at the (   ) in situations.

5 A deep laugh is good for our (   ).

| hospitals / health / humor / techniques / sunshine |

B 音声を聴いて, 次の英文の ( ) 内に適切な語を記入しなさい。

1 The train was late (   ) (   ) the bad weather.

2 He escaped (   ) (   ) a few other prisoners.

3 The thunderstorm lasted (   ) (   ) three hours.

4 Make sure you drink (   ) (   ) water.

5 She (   ) (   ) some spelling errors in my paper.

C 次の日本文に合うように，（　　）内の語句を並べかえて英文を作りなさい。

1 私たちはその川でよく泳いだものだ。
　（the river, swim, to, we, in, used）.

_____

2 それは担当者次第である。
　（who, on, charge, depends, in, it, is）.

_____

3 スミス氏は買い物をしただけでなく食事も作った。
　（also, the meal, only, but, Mr. Smith, shopping, cooked, not, did）.

_____

D 次の英語に相当する日本語を下から選び，記号で答えなさい【症状や徴候②】。

1 hangover （　　）　2 jaundice （　　）　3 swelling （　　）

4 paralysis （　　）　5 coma （　　）　6 sneeze （　　）

7 palpitation （　　）　8 congestion （　　）　9 incontinence （　　）

10 rash （　　）

ア．動悸　イ．くしゃみ　ウ．発疹　エ．二日酔い　オ．失禁
カ．黄疸　キ．うっ血　ク．腫れ　ケ．昏睡　コ．麻痺

Unit 5

Holiday Duty

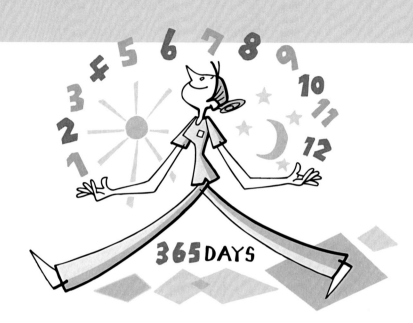

Vocabulary Check

次の日本語に相当する英語を下から選んで記入しなさい。

1 (   )   あきらめ
2 (   )   責任，職務
3 (   )   犠牲
4 (   )   記憶，思い出
5 (   )   同僚
6 (   )   寛大さ
7 (   )   交友，親交
8 (   )   感謝
9 (   )   腫瘍学
10 (   )   宗教

cohort／fellowship／generosity／gratitude／oncology／religion／
reminiscence／resignation／responsibility／sacrifice

Audio

1   A necessary but dreaded duty for most nurses is working on Christmas, Thanksgiving, and other holidays. These traditional family times make being away from home a double hardship, but most nurses attend to their holiday duty with a mix of joy and resignation.

5   First, we realize that if nurses hate to be away from their families on holidays, then patients must feel even worse. Being in the hospital during the time of traditional family gatherings make illness and recovery even more difficult. Many people push themselves to try to be home by Christmas. People who are admitted during the holiday season

10 pin their hopes on being home before festivities begin.

Second, most of us just incorporate holiday duty into our family lives, especially in regard to our children. They are used to hearing that we have to work on weekends sometimes, so they know that mothers and fathers have other responsibilities. Saving lives and caring for sick

15 people is a serious and important matter.

Even young children of nurses can understand that what their parents do is very important and sometimes entails some sacrifice, like having to wait until Mom gets home to open presents or having an evening Thanksgiving dinner so Dad can eat with the family.

Notes

1	dreaded／とても嫌な
2	Thanksgiving／感謝祭の日 (Thanksgiving Day. 米国では11月の第4木曜日)
3	away from ～／～から離れて
3	hardship／苦難
4	attend to ～／～に取り組む
5	hate to ～／～するのを嫌がる
7	gathering／集まり，会合
8	push oneself to ～／～しようと努力する，無理をする
9	admit／入院させる
10	pin one's hope on ～／～に強い期待

をかける，～に希望をつなぐ
10 festivity／(複数形で)祝賀会
11 incorporate A into B／AをBへ組み入れる
12 in regard to ～／～に関しては
12 be used to ～／～に慣れている
13 on weekends／週末に
14 care for ～／～の世話をする，～の面倒を見る
17 entail／伴う
19 so (that) A can ～／Aが～できるように

1   Finally, we rely on our reminiscence of wonderful on-duty holiday
stories. Many involve the sharing of the holiday meal. One nurse told
me that when she and her cohorts saw the holiday schedule and learned
that they were working, they decided they would try to spread a little
5   cheer. They brought in a turkey dinner with all the trimmings for the
families in the waiting room.

Another nurse told me about working in England during the holidays.
Since the patients tend to stay longer in the hospital there, the families
get to know the nurses well. During the holiday season, the families
10   prepared feasts and brought the whole family, distant and near, to the
hospital for a holiday meal. While it was hard to be away from their own
families, the nurses loved the generosity and fellowship of families who
were expressing gratitude to nurses for giving of themselves to benefit
their loved ones.

15   Nurses have joyful stories, like the happy moments of babies born on
Christmas Day to grateful parents who enjoy the greatest gift of all.
Nurses also have sad holiday stories.

One nurse who worked with oncology patients many years ago
related an experience she remembers vividly. She looked me in the eye

Notes

1	rely on 〜／〜を頼りにする	13	benefit／役に立つ，ためになる
1	on-duty／勤務時間中の	14	loved one／最愛の人
2	involve／伴う，関連する	16	grateful／感謝の気持ちを示す
4	spread／広める	18	work with 〜／〜のために働く
5	bring in 〜／〜を持ち込む	18	patient／患者
5	trimming／(複数形で，料理の)添え物，付け合わせ	19	relate／話す，述べる
		19	vividly／鮮やかに
8	tend to 〜／〜する傾向がある	19	look A in the eye／Aの目をじっと見る
9	get to 〜／〜するようになる		
10	feast／ごちそう		

1 and told me the exact date.

"I worked with leukemia patients," she said. "[Back]then, they almost all died. It was the days when hospitals were less user-friendly, and children were strictly banned from visiting. I[was caring for]a 32-year-
5 old man who was dying of leukemia. I asked him what he wanted for Christmas that day and he told me that all he wanted was to see his children. I made a decision I have never regretted."

She went on to relate how she arranged with his wife to bring their three small children to the hospital the next evening. After her strict,
10 rule-enforcing supervisor made rounds, she signaled to the stairwell for the wife to bring in the kids.

She went in his room a few minutes later and found all three children in bed with their dad who had the biggest smile she had ever seen. They showed him pictures, talked about Christmas presents to come,
15 shared those precious moments that only happen between dads and their kids.

The patient died quietly the next morning with his wife at his side. Many years later, my friend is still profoundly moved by this experience. Nurses truly do touch lives.

Notes

1	exact／正確な		8	go on to ～／引き続き～する
2	leukemia／白血病		10	rule-enforcing／規則を守らせる
3	user-friendly／利用者に便利な，使いやすい		10	supervisor／上司
			10	make rounds／巡回する
4	be banned from ～ing／～するのを禁止される		10	signal／合図する
			10	stairwell／階段の吹き抜け
5	die of ～／～が原因で死ぬ		18	be moved／心を動かされる
7	regret／後悔する		18	profoundly／大いに，心から

1   I want to thank my colleagues who give so selflessly of their time and talent during the holidays. It takes a special person to be a nurse. Like our brothers and sisters in the military and the police officer and firefighter ranks who are on duty 365 days a year, we serve because we
5   care. We care about people we don't even know. We care about people whose religion and skin color are different from our own. We care about people whose language we can't understand. Whether it is an important holiday or just a regular Tuesday, nurses are on duty everywhere doing what they do best: caring. Thanks for always being there.

Notes

1	colleague／同僚	4	be on duty／勤務中で
1	give of ～／～を惜しみなく与える	4	serve／役に立つ
1	selflessly／無欲で，利己心を捨てて	5	care about ～／～の世話をする，～の面倒を見る
3	military／軍隊		
3	police officer／警察官	6	be different from ～／～とは異なる
4	firefighter／消防士	7	whether A or B／AであろうとBであろうと
4	rank／階級，身分		

練習問題

A 本文の内容に合うように（　　　）内に入る語を下から選びなさい。

　A nurse worked with （　　　　　　　） patients. One of the patients told the nurse that he wanted to see his （　　　　　　　）. She arranged with his （　　　　　　　） to bring their three small children to the hospital. He smiled when his children showed him （　　　　　　） and talked about Christmas presents. He died quietly the next （　　　　　　） with his wife at his side.

pictures／wife／morning／leukemia／children

B 音声を聴いて，次の英文の（　　　）内に適切な語を記入しなさい。

① She （　　　　　） （　　　　　　　） （　　　　　　　） hard work.

② I （　　　　） （　　　　　） the bus to take me to and from work each day.

③ Tom was （　　　　　） （　　　　　　） old people.

④ Can you look me （　　　　　） （　　　　　　） （　　　　　） and say that?

⑤ The patient （　　　　　） （　　　　　） a heart attack.

C 次の日本文に合うように，（　　　）内の語句を並べかえて英文を作りなさい。

1 彼はナンシーについて調べた。
   （regard, Nancy, he, to, inquiries, in, made）.

_____

2 女性は男性よりも長生きする傾向がある。
   （longer, to, men, live, women, than, tend）.

_____

3 ジョンは車の運転を1年間禁止された。
   （was, a year, banned, driving, John, from, for）.

_____

D 次の英語に相当する日本語を下から選び，記号で答えなさい【疾病や創傷①】。

1 fracture（　　） 2 sprain（　　） 3 arthritis（　　） 4 stroke（　　）

5 tumor（　　） 6 dementia（　　） 7 depression（　　）

8 insomnia（　　） 9 schizophrenia（　　） 10 bulimia（　　）

ア．うつ病　イ．過食症　ウ．不眠症　エ．捻挫　オ．統合失調症
カ．認知症　キ．関節炎　ク．骨折　ケ．脳卒中　コ．腫瘍

Unit 6

Dealing with Reality

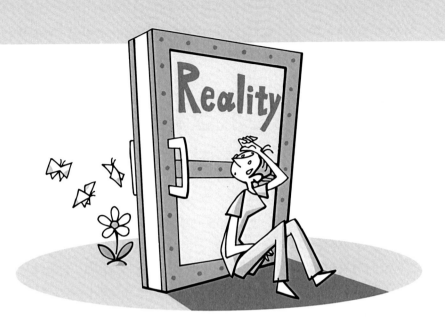

Vocabulary Check

次の日本語に相当する英語を下から選んで記入しなさい。

1 (　　　　　　　　　) 　虚脱感，心身の消耗
2 (　　　　　　　　　) 　絶望
3 (　　　　　　　　　) 　尊厳死
4 (　　　　　　　　　) 　不安，苦悩
5 (　　　　　　　　　) 　将来の展望
6 (　　　　　　　　　) 　場合，時
7 (　　　　　　　　　) 　枯渇，消耗
8 (　　　　　　　　　) 　結果
9 (　　　　　　　　　) 　不便なこと
10 (　　　　　　　　　) 　役に立つもの，値打ちのあるもの

angst ／ burnout ／ commodity ／ depletion ／ despair ／ dignified death ／
inconvenience／occasion／outcome／perspective

1 I recently saw a nurse throw up her hands and declare in an angry, tear-choked voice, "Why in the world did I ever get into nursing?"

 She had just learned she was getting two newly-admitted patients. She already had more to do than she could possibly handle in this
5 lifetime, and she knew it. Call it a sign of the times—doing more with less, too much work and too little time, stress, burnout, anger, despair. Is there any hope?

 Of course there is always hope, but how do we manage these frustrating situations? You've heard of *attitude adjustment*. Then you
10 may be ready for an "expectation adjustment." We were all idealistic and zealous when we became nurses. What happened?

 I am wondering if we can boil it down to an expectation/reality mismatch. It goes something like this: We expected to have time to listen and learn what was really bothering the surgical patient with two
15 little children at home. We expected to make a real positive difference in people's health and happiness.

 The reality, however, is that patient teaching occurs during the four minutes while you are administering your evening medications, when

	deal with 〜／〜に対処する，取り組む
1	throw up one's hands／お手上げだとあきらめる
1	declare／はっきり言う
2	tear-choked／涙にむせぶ
2	in the world／(疑問詞を強調して)いったい全体
2	get into 〜／(業界など)〜に入る
3	newly-admitted／新しく入院した
3	patient／患者
4	handle／対処する，扱う
5	lifetime／生涯
5	a sign of the times／(悪い意味で)時代の象徴，時代を物語るもの
5	do more with less／より少ない労力と時間でより大きな成果をあげる(略語はDMWL)
9	hear of 〜／〜のことを聞く
9	*attitude adjustment*／態度の修正

10	be ready for 〜／〜の準備ができている
10	"expectation adjustment"／「期待の修正」
10	idealistic／理想主義的な
11	zealous／熱心な
12	wonder if 〜／〜かしらと思う
12	boil A down to B／AをBに要約する
13	mismatch／ミスマッチ，食い違い
13	It goes something like this／こんな感じだ
14	bother／悩ます，心配させる
14	surgical／外科の
15	make a difference／影響を与える，重要である
17	The reality is that 〜／現実には〜である
18	administer／投与する
18	medication／薬物，薬剤

1　you really need to be paying attention to right patient, right dose, and the other "rights." The reality is that the only one who listens to the patient's worries about not being able to care for her two small children is the housekeeper. The reality is not what we expected.

5　So do we try to change our expectations or do we try to change the reality? One thing you learn about nurses very quickly is that we do not lower our expectations for our patients. The idealists in us are alive and well. We work to achieve the ideal, whether it is optimal health or a peaceful, dignified death. But I would like to offer a suggestion about

10　our expectations of ourselves.

For some reason, nurses think they are invincible. We think we can and must do everything better and more quickly than anyone else. Faster is better, right? I also have watched the corporate world similarly speed up with some resulting angst and burnout. However,

15　let's face it. In the corporate world, if the two columns on the audit sheet do not add up, no one dies.

Dealing with life and death situations is the factor that skews our vision. Just like police officers who deal with critical situations, we become consumed by the nature of our work. We lose focus of the fact

---

Notes

1	pay attention to ～／～に注意を払う	9	would like to ～／～したい
1	dose／服用量	11	for some reason／どういうわけか
2	"rights"／「正しいこと」	11	invincible／無敵の，不屈の
3	be able to ～／～することができる	13	corporate／企業の
3	care for ～／～の世話をする，～の面倒を見る	14	resulting／結果として生じる
4	housekeeper／(病院の) 清掃係	15	let's face it.／事実として認めよう。
7	lower／下げる，低くする	15	column／(縦の)欄
7	idealist／理想主義者	15	audit sheet／監査シート
7	alive and well／元気で，ぴんぴんして	16	add up／計算が合う
8	work to ～／～するよう努力する	17	skew／歪める
8	achieve／達成する	18	vision／見通す力，展望
8	ideal／理想	18	police officer／警察官
8	whether A or B／AであろうとBであろうと	18	critical／重大な，危機の
8	optimal／最良の，最適の	19	consume／消耗する，使い尽くす
		19	lose focus of ～／～の焦点を失う
		19	the fact that ～／～という事実

1　that not every decision is life and death. If a patient quits breathing, we
react immediately and decisively with the full force of our physical and
emotional selves to save a life. Unfortunately, when the announcement
comes that the parking lot is being repaved and we have to find
5　alternate parking, we often react the same way. We expend a lot of
energy over decisions which are not worthy of the adrenaline drain
they trigger.

　　Perspective is the key. I stand by my sure-fire way of deciding how
much energy to expend on any situation—the five-year test. Before you
10　invest your precious time and energy in any situation, apply the five-
year test: Am I going to remember this in five years? We each have
only so much energy, so let's save it for the truly worthy occasions.
Energy depletion is a major reason we feel the stress, burnout, anger,
and despair mentioned earlier. We are just too tired to deal with it. So,
15　anything that saves our energy is bound to make our lives a little bit
easier and less hectic. Applying the five-year test is an easy way to
save time and energy for the really big decisions.

　　Chances are good that if you give the wrong medication and have a
disastrous outcome, you will remember it forever. So, medication

Notes

1	not every A is ～／すべてのAが～というわけではない	8	sure-fire／絶対確実な
1	quit／やめる	10	invest／費やす
2	immediately／直ちに	10	precious／貴重な
2	decisively／断固として	10	apply／適用する
3	unfortunately／不幸にも	12	only so much／限られた量の
4	repave／舗装しなおす	14	too ～ to...／～すぎて…できない
5	alternate／代わりの	15	be bound to ～／確実に～するはずだ
5	expend／費やす	16	hectic／慌ただしい
6	worthy of ～／～に値する	18	chances are good that ～／～の可能性が高い
6	drain／流出	19	disastrous／悲惨な
7	trigger／引き起こす		
8	stand by ～／～をかたく守る		

administration is a situation worthy of your time and energy. The parking lot situation, however, is not. Yes, it is an inconvenience, a bother, just one more thing; but chances are good that it will **not** become a vivid part of your history. Accept what you cannot change and park somewhere else. Don't worry and fume over it.

One more thing—the pace of healthcare has accelerated. We cannot slow it down or stop it. We cannot control the demands others make of us. But we can control the demands we make of ourselves. If you are not going to remember it in five years, move on. Make a decision, don't second-guess yourself, and leave it in your rearview mirror. Take care of yourself. Nurses are a precious commodity.

練習問題

A 次の英文が，本文の内容と一致する場合にはTを，一致しない場合にはF
を（　　）内に記入しなさい。

（　　）① Nurses are frustrated because they are doing too much work
with too little time.

（　　）② Nurses expected to make a positive difference in people's health
and happiness, but the reality is not what they expected.

（　　）③ Nurses are not idealistic but realistic.

（　　）④ The five-year-test cannot save nurses' time and energy at all.

（　　）⑤ The parking lot situation is an inconvenience for nurses, so they
will remember it forever.

B 音声を聴いて，次の英文の（　　）内に適切な語を記入しなさい。

① I don't know how to（　　　　　）（　　　　　　　）this problem.

② What（　　　　　）（　　　　　　）（　　　　　　）are you talking
about?

③ （　　　　　　）everything（　　　　　）（　　　　　　）the party?

④ Jane asked me what I（　　　　　）（　　　　　）（　　　　　）
do.

⑤ His new book is（　　　　　）（　　　　　）praise.

C 次の日本文に合うように，（　　）内の語句を並べかえて英文を作りなさい。

1. 現実には私たちには家を買う余裕はない。
   (a house, we, afford, is, buy, the reality, to, cannot, that).

_____

2. キャシーは先生の話すことに全く注意を払わなかった。
   (the teacher, paid, to, attention, no, Kathy, said, what).

_____

3. フルートはケースに保管して大切にしなさい。
   (its case, your flute, keeping, of, in, care, by, take, it).

_____

D 次の英語に相当する日本語を下から選び，記号で答えなさい【疾病や創傷②】。

1. pneumonia（　　）2. tuberculosis（TB）（　　）3. bronchitis（　　）

4. asthma（　　）5. heart attack（　　）6. myocardial infarction（　　）

7. hepatitis（　　）8. cystitis（　　）9. anemia（　　）

10. leukemia（　　）

ア．膀胱炎　イ．心筋梗塞　ウ．肝炎　エ．貧血　オ．喘息
カ．肺炎　キ．白血病　ク．気管支炎　ケ．心臓発作　コ．結核

Unit 7

Patient Fears

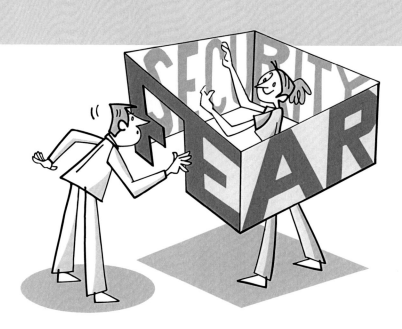

Vocabulary Check

次の日本語に相当する英語を下から選んで記入しなさい。

1 (   )　恐れ，恐怖
2 (   )　わかる，認識する
3 (   )　気づいて，認識のある
4 (   )　吸引
5 (   )　処置
6 (   )　静める，和らげる
7 (   )　説教する，説く
8 (   )　現実
9 (   )　災難，災害
10 (   )　好ましくない，適さない

allay／aware／disaster／fear／hostile／preach／procedure／reality／
recognize／suction

Audio 1

1   I walked through the ICU one day. One patient appeared to have a dozen IV bags hanging and the usual body systems monitor with the cardiac rhythm in plain view. He was on a respirator and had a couple of other machines that I must admit I did not even recognize. I watched

5   the nurse working in that environment, so relaxed, capable, competent, in control, so aware, so ready. It was magical—a scene of total confidence as this very sick man let this nurse hold his life in her hands. I was awed.

   Then I looked again and tried to imagine how this scene appeared to

10   someone who was not a nurse: his wife, his children, his friends. It was probably frightening, the first time they saw someone they loved relying on so many machines, so many bags of medicine. And, I am willing to wager that it probably scared them every time they visited him.

15   For one thing, all that equipment is a reminder of how sick a critical patient is. It is a reminder of just how fragile life can be. But another

Notes

	patient／患者
1	ICU／集中治療室(intensive care unit)
1	appear to～／～と思われる，～のように見える
1	a dozen／多数の
2	IV／点滴，静注 (intravenous)
2	usual／お決まりの，いつもの
2	body system／身体
2	monitor／監視装置，モニター
3	cardiac rhythm／心臓律動
3	in plain view／まる見えで，はっきり見えて
3	respirator／人工呼吸器
3	a couple of～／2, 3の～，いくつかの～
4	admit／認める
5	environment／環境
5	capable／能力のある，熟練した
5	competent／有能な，十分に資格のある
6	in control／(事態を)掌握して，冷静で
6	ready／素早い，敏速な
6	magical／(魔法のように)魅惑的な，

	うっとりさせる
7	confidence／信任，信頼
7	hold ～ in one's hand／～の運命を握っている，～に責任を持つ
8	awe／(通例 be awedで)畏れさせる，畏敬させる
9	try to ～／～してみる
11	frightening／恐ろしい，ぎょっとさせるような
12	rely on ～／～を頼りにする
12	medicine／薬，薬剤
12	be willing to ～／～しても構わない，～するのを厭わない
13	wager／請け合う
13	scare／怖がらせる，おびえさせる
13	every time ～／～するたびに
15	for one thing／(理由の説明に用いて)一つには
15	equipment／器具，装備
15	reminder／思い出させるもの
15	critical／危篤の，重篤な
16	fragile／壊れやすい，もろい

1 aspect of their fear is that this scene is foreign, strange, very complex, and monstrously intimidating. It must be somewhat akin to how I feel when my car will not start. I look under the hood and feel total intimidation and bewilderment. Nothing looks familiar except the
5 radiator where the water goes. Almost everything is unknown to me and causes fear that my ability to get to where I am going depends on something I cannot fix. Family members of patients in the ICU must feel that way about the cardiac rhythm strip—it looks familiar from seeing it on television, but they don't know what it means.

10 Fear must be constant when people are in the ICU. Fear of the unknown, fear of unwanted outcomes, fear of being unable to fix everything. ICU nurses have grown particularly adept at addressing the fears of visitors and patients over the years, but it remains a challenge.

How about the simpler things in hospitals as they relate to patient
15 fears? As we get busier, I worry that we are forgetting the natural fear that patients and families have of the everyday things we do. We used to go into the patient's room *without* the nasogastric tube to explain what gastric suction meant and how it was done. We would explain in

---

Notes

1	aspect／局面，状況	8	strip／（心電図の）データ，細長い紙きれ
1	foreign／異質の，相いれない		
2	monstrously／非常に，ひどく	9	on television／テレビで
2	intimidating／怖い，脅すような	10	constant／絶えず続く，不断の
2	be akin to ～／～と類似している	11	unwanted／望まない，不要な
3	hood／ボンネット	11	outcome／結果，成果
4	intimidation／脅迫，威嚇	12	adept／熟達した
4	bewilderment／当惑，うろたえ	12	address／取り組む，対処する
4	familiar／見慣れている，よく知っている	13	over the years／長年にわたって
		13	remain ～／～のままである
4	except ～／～を除いては	13	challenge／難題，試練
5	radiator／ラジエーター，冷却器	14	How about ～?／～についてはどうか?
5	unknown／知られていない，不明の	14	relate to ～／～に関わる，～に関係する
6	get to ～／～に到着する		
6	depend on ～／～に依存する，～次第である	16	used to ～／かつては～したものだ
		17	nasogastric tube／経鼻胃管
7	fix／直す，修理する	18	gastric／胃部の

1 simple terms and let the patient ask questions. Then we brought in the equipment and in a soothing, soft voice explained every step of the procedure. We stayed with the patient for a few minutes until calmness had returned.

5 　　In these hectic days of doing more with less, I wonder whether we still have the time to leave the tube behind, to recognize and allay patients' fears.

　　How about a simple blood transfusion? Today, people are terrified of having someone else's blood pumped into their veins. They are afraid of 10 the idea, the procedure, and the potential outcomes. I wonder if we recognize that fear and try to reassure the patient; or if we feel lucky to even find the 10 minutes it takes just to get the paperwork done in order to get the blood delivered and the transfusion started?

　　Of course, it's easy for me to sit at this keyboard and preach about 15 the need to spend quality time with our patients, to take the time to reduce their fears and promote their comfort. I haven't just worked 11 hours, my feet don't hurt, and I am not worried that I might get a call in

1   the morning to work for someone who is out with the flu.

    The realities of nursing today are sometimes grim. But I have to hand it to nurses. I still see nurses laughing, caring, explaining, and talking gently and soothingly to frightened patients. You just cannot get a good

5   nurse down. Even when nurses are tired and frustrated, we still take the time to recognize and allay patients' fears of the unknown.

    I think that nurses know that things always get better. We have problems, crises, even disasters—but things always get better. Sharing that ray of hope and confidence is what makes a frightened patient feel

10   the security and confidence that everything will turn out well. I guess when you spend your life taking care of people who are helpless and often hopeless, you insulate yourself against sadness and despair so you can continue to function. The current healthcare crisis is sad and discouraging, but nurses continue to function. In fact, when things get

15   tough is when we often rise to our finest hour.

    I know that nurses will continue to make a difference in people's lives. I hope you will remember that our everyday environment can be a

---

Notes

1	out／(仕事を)休んで		を過ごす
1	flu／インフルエンザ, 流感 (influenza の短縮形)	11	take care of ～／～を世話する
2	grim／厳しい, 気の滅入る	11	helpless／無力な, 自分では何もできない
2	hand／手渡す	12	hopeless／絶望的な, 望みをなくした
4	soothingly／なだめるように	12	insulate／隔離する, 孤立させる
4	get ～ down／～を落ち込ませる, ～をがっかりさせる	12	despair／絶望
5	frustrated／挫折した, 失望した	12	so (that) A can ～／Aが～できるように
5	take the time to ～／～するために時間をさく	13	function／役目を果たす
7	get better／よくなる, 好転する	13	current／現在の
8	crisis／危機, 重大局面	14	discouraging／落胆させる
8	share／共有する	14	in fact／それどころか
9	ray／光線	15	tough／困難な, 辛い
10	security／安全, 安心	15	rise to ～／～に十分応える, ～にうまく対処する
10	turn out ～／結局～になる, ～であることがわかる	15	one's finest hour／最高の瞬間, 栄光の時
10	I guess ～／～と思う	16	make a difference／重要である, 影響を与える
11	spend A (時間) ～ing／～して A (時間)		

1　hostile and frightening place for patients. I implore you to find the time
to answer questions about procedures and spend a few moments just
being present to your patients who trust you enough to place their lives
in your hands. Healthcare can be a fearful place to patients; nurses
5　make it safe.

Notes

1　implore A to ～／Aに～するよう懇
願する
3　present／(ある場所に)いる，存在して

いる
3　place／ゆだねる，任せる

練習問題

A 本文の内容に合うように，次の英文の（ ）内に入る語を下から選びなさい。

The author recognizes that fear must be（ ）when the patients are in the ICU. For one thing, all the equipment reminds us of how sick a critical patient and how（ ）life can be. The author also points out that nurses try to take the time to allay patients' fear of the unknown, fear of the（ ）outcomes. Nurses should make a （ ）patient feel security and（ ）that everything will be all right.

---

confidence／constant／fragile／frightened／potential

B 音声を聴いて，下記英文の（ ）内に適語を記入しなさい。

① I need（ ）（ ）（ ）glasses.

② There was some rioting, but the police are now（ ）（ ）.

③ I（ ）（ ）（ ）（ ）yesterday.

④ I（ ）my wallet（ ）in the kitchen.

⑤ The child（ ）（ ）（ ）dogs.

C 次の日本文に合うように，（ ）内の語句を並べ替えて英文を作りなさい。

1 彼らは週末に勤務しても構わない人たちのリストを持っている。
(are, work weekends, who, a list of people, to, keep, willing, they).

2 よい看護師になるために，一生懸命勉強しなさい。
(in, a good nurse, should, to, you, become, study hard, order).

3 彼女はすべて結局うまくいくだろうと彼らに保証した。
(would, assured, everything, all right, them, out, she, that, turn).

D 次の英語に相当する日本語を下から選び，記号で答えなさい【疾病や創傷③】。

1 mumps （ ）　　2 diabetes （ ）　　3 menopausal disorder （ ）

4 otitis media （ ）　5 cataract （ ）　6 burn （ ）

7 chickenpox （ ）　8 measles （ ）　9 rubella （ ）

10 complication （ ）

> ア．白内障　イ．合併症　ウ．糖尿病　エ．熱傷　オ．風疹
> カ．更年期障害　キ．麻疹，はしか　ク．中耳炎　ケ．水痘
> コ．おたふくかぜ

8 Cultural Differences and Nursing Care

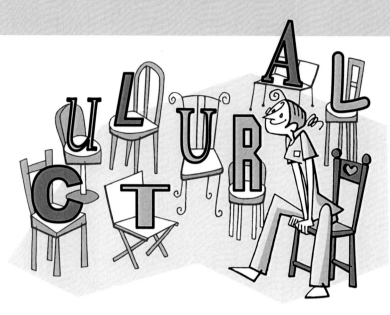

Vocabulary Check

次の日本語に相当する英語を下から選んで記入しなさい。

1 (　　　　　　　　　) 多文化主義
2 (　　　　　　　　　) 雰囲気
3 (　　　　　　　　　) 大多数
4 (　　　　　　　　　) 人種差別
5 (　　　　　　　　　) 性差別
6 (　　　　　　　　　) 年齢差別
7 (　　　　　　　　　) 専門知識
8 (　　　　　　　　　) 局面，状況
9 (　　　　　　　　　) 返答
10 (　　　　　　　　　) 幸福

ageism／aspect／atmosphere／expertise／majority／multiculturalism／
racism／response／sexism／well-being

1   Society appears to be tiring of discussions focused on culture or multiculturalism. And yet, the facts are simple: We are different. We come from different places. We've read from different books and had different experiences. We've heard different lectures and had different

5   role models.

    Some people place value labels on these differences. Deciding on these values, or "judging," creates an atmosphere in which we do not seem to get along very well at all.

    Those of us who have spent the greater part of our nursing careers

10 working with various ethnic groups are equally aware of the differences. But we continue to see the value of peace and harmony, and we have gone on with our work in spite of a society that is color, class, and gender conscious.

    I would like to respectfully and humbly share with you a few hints

15 that have helped me enjoy my nursing career, working with many people who are different from me.

  ◆I have always gone into each setting, no matter how different from my own culture, expecting to be welcomed and accepted. I firmly believe that whatever you expect is what you will find. I expect them to

Notes

1	appear to ～／～のように見える, 思われる	*10*	ethnic／民族の
1	be tiring of ～／～にうんざりしている	*10*	be aware of ～／～に気づいている
		10	equally／同じ程度に, 同様に
1	be focused on ～／～に重点を置かれている	*12*	go on with ～／～を続ける
		12	in spite of ～／～にもかかわらず
2	and yet／それでも, しかもなお	*13*	gender／(社会的・文化的役割としての)性
3	come from ～／～の出身である	*13*	～ conscious／(通例, 複合語で)～の意識の強い, ～を意識した
4	lecture／講義, 訓戒		
5	role model／手本となる人	*14*	would like to ～／～したい
6	place A on B／AをBに置く	*14*	respectfully／謹んで
6	value／価値, 価値観	*14*	humbly／謙虚に
6	label／レッテル	*14*	share／共有する
7	not ～ at all／全く～でない	*17*	go into ～／～の一員となる
7	seem to ～／～のように思われる	*17*	setting／環境, 背景
8	get along／うまくやっていく	*17*	no matter how ～／たとえいかに～であろうとも
9	spend A (時間) ～ing／～してA(時間)を過ごす		
		18	welcome／歓迎する
9	career／職歴, 専門職業	*18*	accept／受け入れる
10	various／様々な	*18*	firmly／断固として
		19	whatever ～／～するものは何でも

1 like me, and I expect to like them and to enjoy my nursing experience with them; and I usually do.

◆Focus on the ways we are alike, not on the ways we are different. I value the confidence Hispanic elders have in their *curanderas* (faith
5 healers).　I admire those elderly black women who spend many hours on Sunday morning and into the afternoon celebrating their love of God at church. I may not do those things, but they do. However, the majority of the things they do are exactly the same things that I do. They worry about their kids. They wonder what to fix for lunch. They try to lose
10 weight. They enjoy fresh flowers. They try to make their money last to the end of the month. So do I. We are all much more alike than we are different. Most of our problems between races, genders, and age groups start when we focus on how we are different.

◆Understand that racism, sexism, and ageism are not exclusive to
15 any one race, any one gender, or any one age group. It was a shock to me to learn that elderly people are sometimes biased against teens or younger people. I have found that racism runs across all races as well. Some people do not realize that multiculturalism includes the culture they are biased against as well as others. When I saw racism and

---

Notes

3	way／観点		
3	alike／同様で，よく似て	*11*	all／全く
4	value／尊重する	*11*	much／(形容詞，副詞の比較級を修飾して) 非常に
4	confidence／信頼		
4	Hispanic／(スペイン語を話す) ラテンアメリカ系の	*12*	most of ～／～の大部分
		12	race／人種
4	elder／年長者	*14*	be exclusive to ～／～だけに限られている
4	*curandera*／(スペイン語) クランデラ (ラテンアメリカの女性民間療法医．祈祷や各種の薬草などを用いる．男性形は*curandero*)	*16*	elderly／年配の
		16	be biased against ～／～に対して偏見を抱いている
4	faith healer／信仰療法を行う人，信仰治療師	*16*	teen／10代の若者
5	admire／賞賛する，敬服する	*17*	run across ～／～に及ぶ
6	celebrate／ほめたたえる	*17*	～ as well／～もまた，なお
8	exactly／まさしく，ちょうど	*18*	some people ～／(後続のothersと呼応して) なかには～な人もいる
8	worry about ～／～を心配する		
9	wonder ～／～だろうかと思う	*18*	include／含む
9	fix／(食事などを) 用意する，作る	*19*	A as well as B／Bはもちろんんも，Bだけでなく A も
10	last／続く		
11	So do I.／(so＋動詞＋主語の形で) 私もそうだ。		

1 ageism across many groups, I learned an important lesson. Bigotry is
not part of anyone's culture. It is a learned personal flaw.

◆Learn about other cultures and share yours. People love to talk
about areas in which they have some expertise, and nothing makes an
5 expert like living an experience. So, go on. Ask people about their
culture. I've noted that nursing students are fairly comfortable with this
aspect. When I ask them, however, if they share their own culture in
return, they look at me as if I have suddenly grown two heads. Don't
assume that others know your culture. Share your experiences, too.

10 ◆For example, ask this question about your patient's culture: "What
did you eat for Sunday dinner when you were growing up?" Black
beans and rice as a response from a patient may sound strange to me,
but my patient may be equally surprised to learn that my family had
fried chicken every Sunday of my youth. It was just a hard and fast
15 rule at our house. Now, most people cannot even remember the last
time they actually fried a piece of chicken. Sharing how my values and
customs have changed over the years, however, shows yet another area
where we share more than we differ.

◆In general, always, always do what you do best—be a caring nurse.

Notes		
1	lesson／教訓	
1	bigotry／頑固な偏見，偏狭な信念	
2	learned／経験によって身についた，後天的な	
2	flaw／欠点	
3	share／伝える	
4	area／領域，分野	
5	expert／専門家	
5	live an experience／実際に経験しながら生きる／	
5	go on／続ける，継続する	
6	note／気づく	
6	fairly／かなり	
6	comfortable／慣れて，不安のない	

7	in return／お返しとして，見返りに	
8	as if 〜／まるで〜であるかのように	
8	grow two heads／頭が二つ生える	
9	assume／当然のことと決めてかかる	
11	grow up／成長する，大人になる	
12	sound／思われる，聞こえる	
14	youth／青年期，青春時代	
14	a hard and fast rule／厳格な規則	
16	actually／実際に	
17	custom／習慣	
17	over the years／長年にわたって	
17	yet another／さらにもう1つの	
19	in general／一般的に	
19	caring／思いやりのある	

1   The language of caring is universal. When you bring love of people and a sincere interest in their well-being into any setting, culture does not matter. You will succeed.

Notes

1   universal／普遍的な，万人共通の   2   sincere／誠実な

1   bring A into B／AをBに加える   3   matter／重要である，問題となる

練習問題

A　本文の内容に合うように，次の英文の（　　）内に入る語を下から選びなさい。

　The author enjoys her nursing（　　　　　），working with many people who are（　　　　）different from hers. She believes herself that most of our problems between races, genders, and age groups take place when we focus on how we are different. When she faced racism and（　　　　）across many different groups, she learned an important lesson. She says that（　　　　）is not part of anyone's culture, but a learned personal（　　　　）.

| ageism／bigotry／career／ethnically／flaw |

B　音声を聴いて，次の英文の（　　）内に適切な語を記入しなさい。

① Mary（　　　　）（　　　　　）be in perfect health.

② The topic today will be（　　　　）（　　　　　）American pop culture.

③ John is（　　　　）（　　　　）well at school.

④ There's nothing to（　　　　）（　　　　）.

⑤ Be nice to others without expecting anything（　　　　）（　　　　）.

C 次の日本文に合うように，（　　　）内の語句を並べかえて英文を作りなさい。

① 私たちは週末のほとんどを家の掃除に費やした。
（cleaning up, of, the house, spent, most, we, the weekend）.

_____

② 彼は彼女の狙っているものに気づいていた。
（of, was, she, what, aiming at, aware, was, he）.

_____

③ 悪天候にもかかわらず私たちはピクニックへ出かけた。
（a picnic, of, went, spite, on, the bad weather, we, in）.

_____

D 次の英語に相当する日本語を下から選び，記号で答えなさい【看護用品や機器】。

① gauze （　　　） ② dressing （　　　） ③ forceps （　　　） ④ scalpel （　　　）

⑤ syringe （　　　） ⑥ tourniquet （　　　） ⑦ defibrillator （　　　）

⑧ ventilator （　　　） ⑨ stethoscope （　　　） ⑩ bedpan （　　　）

ア．聴診器　イ．除細動器　ウ．便器　エ．包帯　オ．人工呼吸器
カ．メス　キ．ガーゼ　ク．注射器　ケ．鉗子　コ．止血帯，圧迫帯

Unit 9

権力闘争

Power Struggle

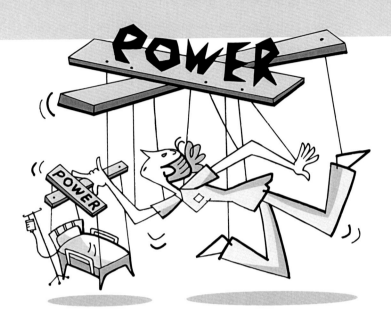

Vocabulary Check

次の日本語に相当する英語を下から選んで記入しなさい。

1. (   ) 施設，組織
2. (   ) 論理
3. (   ) 行動，ふるまい
4. (   ) 医師，内科医
5. (   ) 療法，治療
6. (   ) (湿布などの) 使用
7. (   ) 備品
8. (   ) 職員，スタッフ人員
9. (   ) 倫理
10. (   ) 威厳，尊厳

> application／behavior／dignity／ethics／institution／logic／personnel ／
> physician／supply／therapy

1 Power—it seems like a crazy idea to discuss something such as power in this text, when nurses feel like they have so little of it. However, aren't nurses faced with power struggles every day? Who wins in these cases? And more importantly, are we prepared for these struggles?

5 Power implies that someone has control over someone else. Let's identify who nurses control and who controls us. Then we can decide whether the struggle is worth the effort.

Patients are perhaps the least powerful persons in the hospital, the clinic, or even in their own homes when faced with a healthcare worker. *10* Of course, institutions tell us that the patient is the most important person in the hospital, the reason for our being there, our customer. None of us will argue with that logic, but I still believe that even in the most enlightened, customer-friendly institutions, the patient has almost no power.

15 We tell our patients when to get up, when to eat, even what they can eat, when to get out of bed, and when they can go home. We "restrain" patients whose safety is in jeopardy. We tell 30-year smokers that they cannot smoke in our hospitals and they cannot leave—all for their own good. Then we give them drugs to make our control of their smoking

---

Notes

	power struggle／権力闘争	*5*	have control over 〜／〜を支配している
1	seem like 〜／〜のようである		
1	A such as B／たとえばBのようなA	*6*	identify／特定する，明確にする
2	text／本文，文章	*7*	be worth 〜／〜の価値がある
2	feel like 〜／〜のような気がする	*12*	argue with 〜／〜に反論する，〜と意見が合わない
2	have little of 〜／〜がほとんどない		
3	be faced with 〜／〜に直面している	*13*	enlightened／啓発された，進んだ
		16	"restrain"／「抑制する」
4	be prepared for 〜／〜に対する準備ができている	*17*	in jeopardy／危険にさらされて
5	imply／意味する	*18*	for A's own good／Aのために

56 ■

1　behaviors easier to manage.

　　A vital part of our control over patients is in pain management. Patients do not get pain medication without some input from a nurse. By our charting and our collaboration with physicians, important
5　decisions about pain management and other therapies are made every day.

　　We are experts at controlling families and friends. We tell them where they can park before they even get in the hospital. We tell them when they can visit and how many can come in a room at one time. We also
10　have the ultimate source of control over families and friends: information flow. We can tell them or not tell them whatever we choose.

　　Nurses, however, are also controlled by other people. Ancillary departments, for example, exert great control over nurses' schedules. If a patient is going to have laboratory work done from 9 : 00 AM until
15　noon and will be in physical therapy all afternoon, the assessment, bath, dressing change, and other nursing needs must consequently be done before breakfast.

　　Physicians exert control over nurses by virtue of the nature of the relationship between nurses and physicians. Most actions in hospitals,

2	vital／きわめて重要な	12	ancillary department／補助的な部門（診療科以外の検査や療法を中心とした部門）
2	pain management／疼痛管理		
3	pain medication／鎮痛薬		
3	input／(情報の)提供	13	exert／及ぼす
4	charting／カルテ (chart) を記録すること	14	have laboratory work done／(have A 過去分詞の形で)検査をしてもらう
4	collaboration／協力	15	physical therapy／理学療法
8	get in ～／～の中に入る	15	assessment／アセスメント，評価
9	at one time／同時に，一度に	16	dressing change／包帯交換
10	ultimate／究極の，最後の	16	consequently／結果的に
10	source／源	18	by virtue of ～／～の理由で
10	information flow／情報伝達の流れ		

1 clinics, and home health locations are dependent or interdependent. That means that nurses do not perform the actions without a physician's order. Examples include medication orders or the application of heat or cold.

5 Hospital administration also controls nursing actions by instituting the staffing patterns that directly affect the nurses' ability to do a thorough, professional job of assessment or teaching. Administration controls costs, supplies, personnel, and policies.

So, on the one hand, nurses exert great control over powerless 10 patients, and on the other hand, we are highly controlled by various other persons in the healthcare setting. How do we balance this chaotic approach to our daily schedules?

I believe we all understand the importance of using our ability to control in a helping way, never simply for the pleasure of being in 15 control. When we make decisions that put us in the position of controlling the behavior of others, we must always be sure the decision will benefit them. We must never let our own frustration with those who control us interfere with our judgment regarding the decisions we make for our patients. No matter how tired or frustrated or angry we

Notes

1 home health location／在宅医療の現場
1 dependent／従属関係の，依存の
1 interdependent／相互依存の
2 perform／実行する
5 administration／経営陣，管理者側
5 nursing action／看護行為
5 institute／設ける，制定する
6 staffing pattern／人員配置
6 ability／能力
6 thorough／完全な，徹底的な
9 on (the) one hand／一方では
10 on the other hand／他方では
10 various／さまざまな
11 healthcare setting／保健医療の現場
11 chaotic／混沌とした

12 approach／取り組み方，手法
14 in control／管理して，支配して
15 make a decision／決定する，決断する
16 be sure (that) ～／～ということを確信している
17 benefit／役に立つ，ためになる
17 frustration／フラストレーション，欲求不満
17 those who ～／～な人たち
18 interfere with ～／～を妨げる，じゃまをする
18 regarding ～／～に関しての
19 no matter how ～／どんなに～であろうとも

1   feel, we have to always remember that patients put themselves trustingly in our care. We are bound by duty, morals, ethics, and law to treat them with dignity and professionalism.

    Power is an awesome responsibility. Nurses respect the power we
5   have. We need to use that power to make patients safer and healthier in all clinical settings.

Notes

1	put oneself in 〜／〜に身を置く	2	duty／義務
2	trustingly／信用して	2	moral／(複数形で)道徳
2	be bound by 〜／〜に縛られる, 拘束される	4	awesome／畏怖の念に満ちた
		4	responsibility／責任, 責務

練習問題

A 次の英文が，本文の内容と一致する場合はTを，一致しない場合はFを
（　　　）内に記入しなさい。

（　　）① It is often the cases that nurses take the actions without a doctor's indication.

（　　）② Nurses will only be controlled by physician, but not by hospital administration.

（　　）③ Nurses control over not only their patients but also their families and friends.

（　　）④ Patients are perhaps the least powerful people in the hospital.

（　　）⑤ Nurses have a responsibility to make patients safer and healthier in all clinical settings.

B 音声を聴いて，次の英文の（　　）内に適切な語を記入しなさい。

① I (　　　　　　) fully (　　　　) (　　　　　　) the final exam.

② Their marriage was (　　　　　) (　　　　　) when they noticed.

③ We should do it (　　　　) (　　　　) (　　　　)
(　　　　).

④ He had to work harder (　　　　) (　　　　) (　　　　)
his position.

⑤ Her family problems began to (　　　　　) (　　　　) her work.

C 次の日本文に合うように，（　　　）内の語句を並べかえて英文を作りなさい。

[1] フラストレーションがたまっていたので，彼女は一度に3つのクッキーをつまんだ。
(time, three cookies, feeling, at, took, frustrated, she, one).

_____

[2] どんなに一生懸命やってもその箱を開けることができない。
(I, how, the box, try, hard, can't open, matter, I, no).

_____

[3] 何人もその古い基準に拘束されるものではない。
(shall, be, no, by, the old standards, one, bound).

_____

D 次の英語に相当する日本語を下から選び，記号で答えなさい【診療科】。

[1] surgery（　　　）[2] urology（　　　）[3] gynecology（　　　）

[4] pediatrics（　　　）[5] obstetrics（　　　）[6] dermatology（　　　）

[7] psychiatry（　　　）[8] orthopedics（　　　）[9] ophthalmology（　　　）

[10] internal medicine（　　　）

ア．皮膚科　イ．内科　ウ．精神科　エ．眼科　オ．整形外科
カ．小児科　キ．外科　ク．泌尿器科　ケ．産科　コ．婦人科

Unit 10 Attitude is Everything!

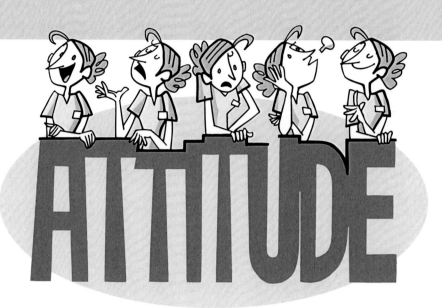

Vocabulary Check

次の日本語に相当する英語を下から選んで記入しなさい。

1 (	)	態度，心構え
2 (	)	熟考する
3 (	)	話題にする，言及する
4 (	)	大目に見る，許容する
5 (	)	忍耐，辛抱強さ
6 (	)	見解，見地
7 (	)	健全な，有益な
8 (	)	（意味・感情などを）伝える
9 (	)	（援助などを）する，与える
10 (	)	求人，人材募集

attitude／convey／healthy／mention／outlook／patience／ponder／
recruitment／render／tolerate

1   In my speaking opportunities, one of my favorite topics is attitude. I love to share *the Family Circus* cartoon in which Billy and Dolly are both contemplating a rose. With a scowl, Billy grumbles at the fact that roses have thorns. Dolly, however, gleefully sings her happiness that
5   thorns have roses!

At the bottom of this cartoon, I have written the words, "Attitude is everything!" I keep it prominently displayed on my bulletin board for my students to ponder.

It seems strange to me to have to tell someone that attitude is
10   important. It seems so self-evident, it may be ridiculous to even mention. But if that is true, why do we encounter so many people with bad attitudes?

I no longer give the benefit of the doubt in this matter. I used to say, "Oh, she is just having a bad day," or, "I must have caught her at an
15   inopportune moment," or some other excuse. Not anymore. I do not excuse and cannot tolerate bad attitudes. Life is too short and the world is too needy to have to tolerate someone who is diligently working to

Notes

1	opportunity／機会	10	ridiculous／ばかげた
1	favorite／特に好きな	11	encounter／出会う
2	share／共有する	13	no longer ～／もはや～でない
2	*the Family Circus*／『ザ・ファミリー・サーカス』(米国の漫画家 Bill Keane と Jeff Keane による，1コマで一般家庭の生活を表現した新聞連載漫画)	13	give the benefit of the doubt／疑わしい点を善意に解釈する
		13	in this matter／この件に関して
		13	used to ～／かつては～したものだ
2	cartoon／(新聞などの)時事漫画	14	have a bad day／ついてない日だ
3	contemplate／熟視する	14	at an inopportune moment／折悪く，都合の悪いときに
3	scowl／しかめっつら		
3	grumble at ～／～についてぶつぶつ言う	15	excuse／弁解，言い訳
		15	Not anymore.／もはやそうではない。今ではそうじゃない。
3	the fact that ～／～という事実		
4	thorn／(植物の)トゲ	16	excuse／弁解する，言い訳する
4	gleefully／陽気に	17	too ～ to ...／…するには～すぎる，あまりにも～なので…できない
6	at the bottom of ～／～の下部に		
7	keep／ずっと(ある状態に)しておく	17	needy／貧乏な，貧困の(ここでは口語で「他人に頼ってばかりの」「過度に依存する」といった意味)
7	prominently／目立つように		
7	bulletin board／掲示板		
9	seem／思われる	17	diligently／熱心に，こつこつと
10	self-evident／自明の		

1 make things worse. I simply have no patience for these bad-attitude people anymore.

In healthcare, a positive attitude is vital. You cannot realistically expect sick people to always have a happy outlook or a positive attitude.

5 Therefore, the attitude of the nurse is even more vital to a healthy outcome. Be careful, though! An over-the-top bright and cheery approach is not the answer either. Sometimes, too much cheer is as bad as too little. The answer here, then, is in a basic expectation that things will go well.

10 Nurses must convey a positive attitude when working with our patients. We must expect that the patient will do well. We must share that expectation with the person and family. We must appear glad to be at the patient's bedside (whether we are or not), and that patient should feel like the most important person in the world because of our

15 attention and caring. If we are complaining about being short-staffed, about being short-changed in the cafeteria line, or about how much we pay in taxes, the patient will be hard pressed to believe we really care about the situation at hand. An important part of the art of nursing is making the patient the center of our universe when we are rendering

Notes

1	no 〜 anymore／今はもう〜でない	12	be at A's bedside／Aの枕元に付き添う
3	positive／積極的な，前向きの		
3	vital／きわめて重要な	13	whether 〜 or not／〜であろうとなかろうと
3	realistically／現実的には		
4	expect／期待する	14	because of 〜／〜のおかげで，〜の理由で
5	therefore／それゆえ		
6	outcome／結果，成果	15	attention／世話，手当て
6	though／(通例，文尾で) でも，もっとも	15	complain about 〜／〜について不平を言う
6	over-the-top／過度の，極端な		
6	cheery／陽気な	15	short-staffed／人手不足の
7	approach／取り組み方	16	short-changed／つり銭をごまかされた
7	not 〜 either／〜もまた〜でない	17	tax／税金
7	cheer／陽気，元気	17	be hard pressed to 〜／〜するのは難しい，〜するのに苦労する
8	expectation／期待		
9	go well／うまくいく，順調に進む	17	care about 〜／〜に関心がある，〜を気にする
10	work with 〜／〜のために働く		
11	do well／回復する，よくなる	18	at hand／目の前にある，目下の
11	share A with B／AをBと共有する	18	art／技術

1　care.

　A positive attitude is vital when working with other people besides patients as well. Coworkers have problems of their own, problems that you probably would just as soon not have to share. Your positive
5　attitude, however, might just help them get through at least one shift with a little less stress and a bit more positive energy.

　Another important aspect of having a positive attitude is its effect on your personal achievement. To get ahead in life, we all need a little help. Think about it. Recruitment and retention strategies occupy a large
10　amount of the hospital administration's time. When they make retention or promotion decisions, it is just smart business to select the person with a positive attitude since that person will contribute to the type of work setting that makes people want to come to work and stay there. A positive attitude can be a career booster, and a negative attitude can be
15　a career buster.

　So, is attitude important? No—it is vital! A healthy attitude tells the world that not only do you like them, but you like yourself as well. There is no greater gift you can give than to make someone's day a little brighter. And the funny thing is, the more you give away

Notes

2	besides ～／～に加えて，～のほかに	9	a large amount of ～／多くの～
3	～ as well／～もまた，同様に	10	administration／管理部門，経営陣
3	coworker／同僚	10	make a decision／決定する
3	A of one's own／自分自身のA	11	promotion／昇進，昇格
5	get through／やり終える，済ます	11	smart／賢明な，賢い
5	at least／少なくとも	11	business／仕事，業務
5	shift／(交替制の)勤務時間	12	contribute to ～／～に貢献する
6	a bit／(比較級を修飾して)ちょっと，少し	13	work setting／労働環境，職場環境
7	aspect／局面，状況	14	career／経歴，職歴
7	effect／効果，影響	14	booster／後押し役，推進するもの
8	achievement／業績，達成	15	buster／破壊役，ダメにするもの
8	get ahead／出世する，成功する	17	not only A but (also) B／AだけでなくBもまた
9	retention／(人材)確保，維持	19	the more ～, the more ～／(the 比較級 ～, the 比較級…の形で) ～すればするほど，いっそう…する
9	strategy／戦略，方策		
9	occupy／占める，(労力などを)必要とする	19	give away／(無償で)与える，提供する

1 happiness and kindness, the more it comes right back to you.

I challenge you to consciously go out today and make this world a little brighter. You will be surprised how good you, and others, feel.

Notes	

2 challenge A to 〜／Aに〜するよう にあえて要求する

2 consciously／意識的に，故意に
2 go out／外へ出る，出かける

練習問題

A 次の英文が，本文の内容と一致する場合はＴを，一致しない場合はＦを
（　　）内に記入しなさい。

（　　）① Nothing is more important for nurses than positive attitude.
（　　）② A positive attitude is vital for a nurse to find faults with other coworkers.
（　　）③ Nurses should make the patients the center of their work.
（　　）④ The author cannot put up with a person who behaves bad attitudes.
（　　）⑤ A bright and cheery approach is of great importance to make the patients feel good.

B 音声を聴いて，下記英文の（　　）内に適語を記入しなさい。

① Look at the figure （　　　　　）（　　　　　　）（　　　　　　）

（　　　　　　） the page.

② Sorry, but this application is （　　　　　）（　　　　　　） available

for download.

③ Jesse didn't （　　　　　）（　　　　　　） what other people said to

him.

④ I was able to successfully （　　　　　）（　　　　　　） my

assignment and hand it in on time.

⑤ Have you （　　　　　）（　　　　　　）（　　　　　　） yet?

C 次の日本文に合うように，（　　　）内の語句を並べ替えて英文を作りなさい。

1　そのスーツケースは一人で運ぶには重すぎた。
　（heavy, too, the suitcase, alone, carry, to, was）.

_____

2　ハリーは自分自身の会社をはじめるために退社した。
　（own, a business, to, left the company, of, start, his, Harry）.

_____

3　勉強すればするほど物知りになる。
　（you, better, study, the, know, the, you, more）.

_____

D 次の英語に相当する日本語を下から選び，記号で答えなさい【看護師】。

1　circulating nurse（　　）　2　clinical nurse specialist（CNS）（　　）

3　head nurse（＝nurse manager）（　　）

4　licensed practical nurse（LPN）（　　）

5　nurse midwife（　　）　6　nurse anesthetist（　　）

7　public health nurse（＝community health nurse）（　　）

8　registered nurse（RN）（　　）　9　scrub nurse（　　）

10　charge nurse（　　）

ア．看護助産師，助産師　イ．麻酔専門看護師　ウ．看護師長
エ．主任看護師　オ．（手術室）間接介助看護師，外回り看護師
カ．（手術室）直接介助看護師，器械出し看護師　キ．臨床専門看護師
ク．有資格実務看護師　ケ．地域保健看護師，保健師　コ．登録看護師

Unit 11

Student Nurses— Investing in the Future

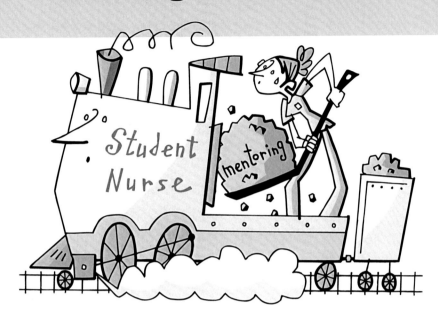

Vocabulary Check

次の日本語に相当する英語を下から選んで記入しなさい。

1	(	)	投資する
2	(	)	挑戦，課題
3	(	)	指導する，導く
4	(	)	ケア提供者
5	(	)	兆候
6	(	)	(負債・損失などを) 負う
7	(	)	感謝
8	(	)	相談，協議
9	(	)	憤慨して，腹を立てて
10	(	)	改正する，直す

appreciation ／ caregiver ／ challenge ／ consultation ／ incur ／ indication ／
invest ／ mentor ／ rectify ／ upset

Audio 1

Now, an important topic about our future—nursing students. There has been a huge shift in the minds and hearts of nurses regarding student nurses over the past few years, from a positive approach to a more negative one. I think this shift has been unconscious and perhaps

5 even unwanted. Nevertheless, this change in thinking is out there in plain view, and it needs to be addressed.

First, we all agree that being a nursing student is an enormous challenge. For years, nurses have welcomed their role in developing and mentoring students. It was a source of pride and self-indulgence

10 to contribute in a meaningful way to a student's education. We looked at them as our future colleagues and perhaps our replacements as we moved on to bigger and better things. We also saw in them our own caregivers as we aged, so we selfishly wanted high-quality nurses who were almost as good as we were. Something, however, has

15 changed.

Nurses who once were eager to have a student assigned to them now

---

Notes

	student nurse／看護学生，見習い看護師(主に，病院での「看護実習生」を意味する)	6	address／取り組む，対処する
		7	enormous／大変な，ものすごい
1	nursing student／看護学生(主に，大学や専門学校で「看護学を学ぶ学生」を意味する)	8	for years／何年も
		8	welcome／喜んで受け入れる
2	huge／巨大な，莫大な	8	role／役割
2	shift／転換，変化	9	self-indulgence／わがまま，身勝手
2	in the minds and hearts of ～／～の心の中で，精神面で	10	contribute to ～／～に貢献する
		10	meaningful／有意義な
2	regarding ～／～に関して，～の点では	11	colleague／同僚
		11	replacement／交替要員，後任者
3	over the past few years／この数年で	12	move on to bigger and better things／よい仕事につく，社会的地位が高くなる
3	positive／積極的な，前向きの		
3	approach／取り組み方	13	age／年を取る
4	negative／消極的な，悲観的な	13	selfishly／自分本位に，利己的に
4	unconscious／自覚しない，無意識の	13	high-quality／質の高い
5	unwanted／望まない，不要な	14	almost／ほとんど
5	nevertheless／それにもかかわらず	14	as ～ as A／Aと同じくらい～な
5	out there／世の中に，目につくところに	16	be eager to ～／しきりに～したがる
5	in plain view／まる見えで，はっきり見えて	16	have a student assigned／(have A 過去分詞の形で)学生を割り当ててもらう
6	need to ～／～する必要がある		

1 hide at the end of the hall, hoping not to be noticed when the instructor approaches. Even the most patient mentors are requesting limited time with students.

From all indications, nurses would rather just give medications
5 themselves than watch a student prepare the drugs. Why? What has happened? Are today's students suddenly much less talented? Have the faculty stopped teaching?

Truthfully, it appears that students and the faculty have remained relatively the same. What has changed is the practice environment.
10 Nurses are being asked to do more with less. We have all seen and heard discussions about this situation, but what does it really mean when it comes to student mentoring?

Doing more with less means caring for sicker and sicker patients on the general medical-surgical units, for example. Today's typical medical-
15 surgical patient would have been a typical ICU patient just a few short years ago; but ICU is expensive, and the goal has become to get the patient out as quickly as possible without incurring high costs.

Doing more with less means attracting a decreasing number of

Notes

1	hide／隠れる	10	do more with less／より少ない労力と時間でより大きな成果を上げる
1	at the end of ～／～の端に		
1	hall／廊下	12	when it comes to ～／～について言えば
1	notice／気づく		
1	instructor／指導者，教員	13	care for ～／～の世話をする，～の面倒を見る
2	even ～／～でさえ		
2	request／頼む，要請する	13	sicker and sicker／(比較級 and 比較級の形で) ますます具合の悪い
2	limited time／限られた時間		
4	would rather A than B／BよりもむしろAしたい	14	general medical-surgical units／一般の内科・外科病棟
4	medication／薬，薬剤	14	for example／たとえば
6	talented／有能な，才能のある	14	typical／典型的な
7	faculty／(大学の)教授陣	15	ICU／集中治療室 (intensive care unit)
8	truthfully／正直なところ	16	get ～ out／～を追い出す，～を外に出す
8	it appears that ～／～と思われる		
8	remain ～／～のままである	17	as ～ as possible／できるだけ～
9	relatively／比較的に	18	attract／引きつける
9	practice environment／実習環境	18	a decreasing number of ～／ますます少ない数の～
10	ask A to ～／Aに～するように頼む，求める		

1　unlicensed assistive personnel to the field who have less qualifications and abilities. And the reason? The computer industry is begging for employees who can read, write, and think—and it pays attractive salaries. We pay unlicensed assistive personnel low wages, ask them to
5　do menial tasks, and often show them little appreciation. Many have moved on to greener pastures in other industries, leaving us short-handed in hospitals. This change in staffing mix means that nurses must often do low-skill tasks along with all of the other expected responsibilities.

10　　Doing more with less means fewer nurses on each unit for consultation, collaboration, and support. Many hospitals have stripped nursing units to the bone in order to decrease costs. The result—a preponderance of poor outcomes, such as falls and pressure sores, linked to low ratios of registered nurses. Administrators are now hearing from
15　more patients, families, and physicians who are becoming upset and frustrated with the situation. Therefore, hospitals are attempting to rectify this short-sighted action, but the return of nurses to the hospital is slow, and students are paying the price.

Notes

1	unlicensed／免許を持っていない	12	in order to ～／～するために
1	assistive personnel／補助職員	12	cost／費用，経費
1	field／分野	13	preponderance／圧倒的多数
1	qualification／資格，能力	13	outcome／結果，成果
2	beg for ～／～請う，～を頼む	13	A such as B／たとえばBのようなA
4	wage／賃金，労賃	13	fall／(患者の)転倒
5	menial／つまらない，卑しい	13	pressure sore／褥瘡，床ずれ
5	task／仕事，職務	13	link to ～／～とつながる
6	move on to ～／～へ移動する	14	ratio／比率
6	greener pastures／より青い牧草地 （ここでは「より魅力的な職場」を指す）	14	registered nurse／登録看護師
		14	administrator／管理者
6	leave us short-handed／(leave A Bの 形で)私たちを人手不足の状態にして おく	14	hear from ～／～から話を聞く，～ の意見を聞く
		16	frustrated／いら立った，失望した
7	staffing mix／多職種連携	16	therefore／それゆえ
8	along with ～／～に加えて	16	attempt to ～／～しようと企てる， 試みる
9	responsibility／責任，責務		
11	collaboration／協働，協力	17	short-sighted／近視眼的な，先見の 明がない
11	strip／取り去る，取り除く		
12	to the bone／徹底的に，最小限度まで	18	pay the price／代償を払う，つけが回る

In summary, why don't nurses want to work with students? They are too tired, too overworked, and too busy. They have more than they can handle with their own patients and expected responsibilities. If time allowed, however, I believe most nurses still want to work with students.

Don't get me wrong. Faculty members have the obligation to prepare students to provide care. Students cannot learn solely on the job; they must know a great deal from laboratory practice before they ever set foot on the nursing unit. Together, however, faculty and professional nurses can provide a meaningful experience for the student and a safe experience for the patient; faculty must be attentive to student needs while nurses are attentive to patient needs.

We cannot give up on educating future nurses. We need them now more than ever; but this education is a cooperative process. Everyone— the nurse, the faculty, and especially the student—must take responsibility for making the experience effective. Tomorrow's healthcare system depends on it.

Notes

1	in summary／要するに
2	overworked／過労の，働きすぎの
3	handle／対処する，扱う
3	if time allowed／時間があれば
6	Don't get me wrong.／誤解しないでください。
6	obligation／義務
7	provide／提供する
7	solely／単に
7	on the job／仕事中に，仕事をして
8	a great deal／たくさん，多量
8	laboratory practice／実習室での練習

8	set foot on ～／～に足を踏み入れる
11	be attentive to ～／～に配慮する，～に気を配る
13	give up on ～／～を断念する，～に見切りをつける
14	more than ever／ますます，これまで以上に
14	cooperative／協働の，助け合う
14	process／作業，行為
16	effective／効果のある，有効な
17	depend on ～／～次第である，～にかかっている

練習問題

A 本文の内容に合うように，次の英文の（　　）内に入る語を下から選びなさい。

Nowadays nurses are not (　　　　　) to mentor students. The main reason is that nurses are being asked to do (　　　　　) with (　　　　　). They have to (　　　　　) for sicker and sicker patients than before. They cannot have enough (　　　　　) personnel because of the advent of a more attractive workplace: the computer industry. Moreover, many hospitals have decreased the number of (　　　　　). Therefore, nurses are too (　　　　　), too overworked, and too busy to (　　　　　) student nurses.

assistive／care／eager／educate／less／more／nurses／tired

B 音声を聴いて，下記英文の（　　）内に適語を記入しなさい。

1 The construction plan has changed (　　　　　) the (　　　　　) (　　　　　) (　　　　　).

2 I (　　　　　) (　　　　　) stay in (　　　　　) go out in the rain.

3 Anna decided to (　　　　　) (　　　　　) (　　　　　) another job that would advance her career.

4 The company cut the number of employees (　　　　　) (　　　　　) (　　　　　).

5 The last time Jack (　　　　　) (　　　　　) (　　　　　) that house was 30 years ago.

C 次の日本文に合うように，（　　）内の語句を並べ替えて英文を作りなさい。

① 顧客からの苦情には迅速に対処する必要がある。
（need, quickly, we, address, to, complaints, customer）.

② 水泳について言えば，マークが一番だ。
（it, is, to, when, the best, Mark, comes, swimming）.

③ 冬場はできるだけ慎重な運転をこころがけてください。
（as, drive, in winter, please, carefully, possible, try to, as）.

D 次の英語に相当する日本語を下から選び，記号で答えなさい【薬剤】。

① antibiotic（　　）　② decongestant（　　）　③ antacid（　　）

④ sedative（　　）　⑤ antidepressant（　　）　⑥ antihypertensive（　　）

⑦ suppository（　　）　⑧ ointment（　　）　⑨ laxative（　　）

⑩ NSAID（　　）

| ア．軟膏　イ．坐薬　ウ．緩下薬，通じ薬　エ．非ステロイド系抗炎症薬 |
| オ．抗うつ薬　カ．充血除去薬，うっ血除去薬　キ．鎮静薬 |
| ク．抗高血圧症薬　ケ．制酸薬　コ．抗生物質 |

Unit 12

Graduation—Nursing Beginnings

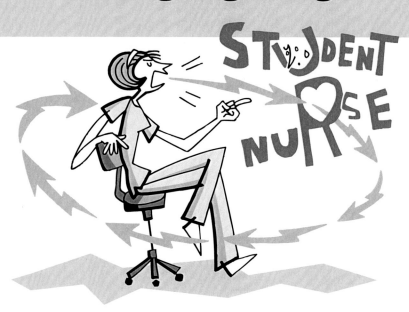

Vocabulary Check

次の日本語に相当する英語を下から選んで記入しなさい。

① (　　　　　　　　) 感謝に満ちた
② (　　　　　　　　) 神聖な
③ (　　　　　　　　) 熱意にあふれた
④ (　　　　　　　　) 現在の
⑤ (　　　　　　　　) 自分を主張する
⑥ (　　　　　　　　) 複雑な
⑦ (　　　　　　　　) 挫折感を抱かせる
⑧ (　　　　　　　　) 思いやりのある
⑨ (　　　　　　　　) 快適そうな，居心地のよさそうな
⑩ (　　　　　　　　) 安心させる

assertive／compassionate／complex／current／enthusiastic／frustrating／
grateful／hallowed／reassuring／welcoming

1 Graduation from nursing school is a wonderful experience. Grateful relief that the rigors of the formal education process are complete and eager enthusiasm to begin a new career are just some of the emotions that new nurses experience.

5 A whole new crop of nurses emerges from the hallowed halls of nursing schools. They are a welcome sight. These enthusiastic new nurses join a tired nurse population. Nurses in hospitals, where most of the new graduates get their first jobs, are feeling the pinch of the nursing shortage, so each new class of graduates are welcomed with

10 open arms by the current nursing workforce.

What will these new nurses find? Will they find a mentor who is happy to show them the ropes, to share insights, to offer support when the first problem arises? Or will they find seasoned nurses who are too tired to help, stretched too thin to offer the moral support they need, or

15 who have the attitude, "I learned the hard way, now you learn the hard way."

I believe that emerging nurses are a fragile commodity. I think they must be handled with care. I can hear my experienced colleagues

Notes

1	graduation／卒業	*10*	workforce／人員，全職員
2	relief／安心，安堵感	*11*	mentor／指導者
2	rigor／厳しさ	*12*	show 〜 the ropes／〜にこつを教える
2	complete／終了した		
3	enthusiasm／熱意	*12*	insight／深い理解，見識
3	emotion／感情	*12*	offer／提供する，申し出る
5	whole／全く	*13*	arise／生じる
5	crop／群れ，集団	*13*	seasoned／経験豊かな，熟練した
5	emerge／現れる	*13*	too 〜 to …／〜すぎて…できない
6	welcome／喜ばしい	*14*	stretched thin／精神的に参っている
6	sight／光景	*14*	moral support／精神的な支援
7	join／合流する，加わる	*15*	attitude／態度
7	tired／疲れた	*15*	the hard way／苦労して
7	population／集団	*17*	emerging／現れたばかりの，新人の
8	graduate／卒業生	*17*	fragile／壊れやすい，もろい
8	pinch／苦しい状況	*17*	commodity／役に立つもの
9	shortage／不足	*18*	handle 〜 with care／〜を注意して扱う
9	class／同期生		
9	with open arms／心から喜んで	*18*	colleague／同僚

¹ sighing under their breaths and muttering something about, "What makes them so special? No one gave me special treatment."

Many nurses have long memories. We remember every slight, every snub, every rude word that was ever uttered by a thoughtless

⁵ supervisor or an abrasive colleague. We take it personally, and we vow to get even. Then, unfortunately, we often strike out at the person we view as dependent or less powerful than we are. That person is often the new kid on the block, the new graduate. At a time when they need nurturing and support, we often use them as a way to get even for all of

¹⁰ the grief we have suffered over the years. It feels so good to finally "get even." But I want to point out the risk with this type of abusive behavior.

Previously, if the new graduate could not take it, they would leave. That way, only the fittest and the strongest survived in the busy

¹⁵ hospital environment. It was really not a problem; we would just get another new student who was probably stronger anyway. The problem is that today, the applicant pool is diminishing. There aren't long lines of other students waiting for that job. If we run off the new graduates who

---

Notes

1	sigh／ため息をつく	*8*	the new kid on the block／新入り
1	under one's breath／小声で	*9*	nurturing／育成，育てること
1	mutter／つぶやく	*9*	way／手段
2	treatment／扱い	*10*	grief／苦しみ
3	have long memories／ずっと前のことを覚えている	*10*	suffer／(不快なことを)経験する，苦しむ
3	slight／軽蔑，無礼	*10*	over the years／長年にわたって
4	snub／冷遇，無視	*11*	point out／指摘する
4	rude／無礼な	*11*	abusive／虐待的
4	utter／口に出す	*12*	behavior／ふるまい，行動
4	thoughtless／思いやりのない	*13*	previously／以前は
5	supervisor／上司	*13*	take／耐える，我慢する
5	abrasive／いらいらさせるような	*14*	that way／そんなふうに
5	take ～ personally／～を個人への当てつけとして受け取る	*14*	the fittest／最も環境に適応した者
5	vow to ～／～することを誓う	*14*	survive／生き残る
6	get even／仕返しをする	*15*	environment／環境
6	unfortunately／不運にも	*16*	anyway／とにかく
6	strike out at ～／～に打ってかかる	*17*	applicant／志願者，候補者
7	view A as B／AをBとみなす	*17*	pool／要員
7	dependent／依存している	*17*	diminish／減少する
		18	run off／追い出す

are somewhat insecure or who fail to be assertive from the first day on the job, we run the risk of having no one to share the complex duties of the work environment.

The environment that the new graduate of today is entering is vastly different than the one we encountered during our first month as a new nurse. The patients are sicker, the machines are more complex, the pace is faster, and the supportive nurturing colleague is harder to find. It can be overwhelming. Professional nursing cannot afford to invest two to three years in the education of a nurse only to find that after a frustrating first year, this nurse decides to get into another field. When nurses leave, not one patient benefits. Other nurses suffer because they must now pick up the slack.

How can nurses present a compassionate and welcoming environment for new nurses? How can we assure that they will thrive and prosper in their new career?

Smile at them. Tell them you remember what it was like. Share some anecdote about how you did similar things when you were a new nurse. You are a hero to them, an icon, a person of such high esteem that they can never hope to be as experienced and competent. Let them into your

Notes

1	somewhat／やや，いくぶん
1	insecure／不安な，自信のない
1	fail to ～／～できない
2	run the risk of ～／～の危険を冒す
2	duty／職務
4	be different than ～／～とは異なっている (from ではなく than を使うのは主に《米》)
4	vastly／非常に
5	encounter／出会う
7	supportive／支えとなってくれる
7	nurture／教育する，養成する
8	overwhelming／どうしようもない，抵抗できないくらいひどい
8	professional／専門職の
8	cannot afford to ～／～する余裕がない
8	invest／投資する，使う
9	only to ～／結局～するだけの結果になる
10	field／分野
11	not one ～／ただ1人の～もない
11	benefit／得をする，恩恵を受ける
12	pick up the slack／代わりを務める，不足を補う
13	present／差し出す，渡す
14	assure／保証する，断言する
14	thrive／成長する
14	prosper／成功する
16	share／伝える，話す
17	anecdote／逸話，エピソード
17	similar／よく似た，同類の
18	icon／憧れの的，偶像
18	such ～ that...／とても～なので…である
18	esteem／尊敬
19	competent／有能な
19	let A into B／AにBを打ち明ける

■79

1 　real self. Invest a little time with them. I remember being scared to
　　death, and I remember how much a reassuring smile meant to me.
　　　We have to transform the nursing environment into a safe, secure,
　　and welcoming place for new nurses, or they will go elsewhere to find
5 　one. When you invest in a new nurse, you improve the future for both
　　of you.

Notes

1　self／自己，自分の本質　　　　　　3　secure／安心していられる
1　scared／おびえた，こわがった　　　4　or／(命令文などの後で)さもなければ
1　to death／死ぬほど，ひどく　　　　5　improve／向上させる
3　transform A into B／AをBに変える

練習問題

A 次の英文が，本文の内容と一致する場合にはTを，一致しない場合にはF
を（　　）内に記入しなさい。

（　　）① New graduates are welcomed by nurses in hospitals because of nursing shortage.

（　　）② Emerging nurses are tough and have no need for special consideration.

（　　）③ It isn't a big problem even if new nurses give up the nursing career easily.

（　　）④ The working environment for nurses today is more stressful than ever before.

（　　）⑤ A little time invested with new nurses will help them stay in nursing profession.

B 音声を聴いて，次の英文の（　　）内に適切な語を記入しなさい。

① The rare book must be （　　　　　）（　　　　　）（　　　　　）.

② The young girl sighed （　　　　　）（　　　　　）（　　　　　）.

③ His comments （　　　　　）（　　　　　）（　　　　　） valuable.

④ Are you ready to （　　　　　）（　　　　　）（　　　　　）

（　　　　　） losing everything?

⑤ The movie scared the boys （　　　　　）（　　　　　）.

C 次の日本文に合うように，（　　　）内の語句を並べかえて英文を作りなさい。

1. 私たちにはそのような高級車を買う余裕はない。
   （to, a luxury car, we, buy, cannot, such, afford）.

   _____

2. 私は家に走って戻ったが，誰もいなかった。
   （stayed there, that, my house, to, I, no one, find, only, ran back to）.

   _____

3. 急がないと始発電車に乗り遅れるよ。
   （train, miss, up, first, you'll, hurry, the, or）.

   _____

D 次の英語に相当する日本語を下から選び，記号で答えなさい【略語】。

1. OR （　　） 2. ICU （　　） 3. CC （　　） 4. STD （　　）

5. CPR （　　） 6. SIDS （　　） 7. SOB （　　） 8. ADL （　　）

9. ENT （　　） 10. Rx （　　）

ア．日常生活動作　イ．心肺蘇生術　ウ．息切れ　エ．処方箋
オ．集中治療室　カ．性感染症　キ．手術室　ク．耳鼻咽喉科
ケ．主訴　コ．乳幼児突然死症候群

Unit 13

Lifelong Learning— A Nursing Commitment

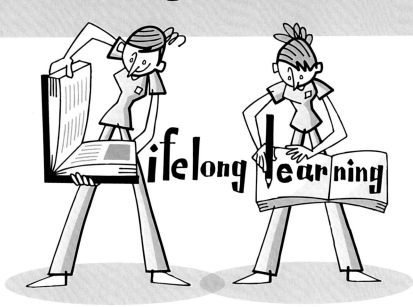

Vocabulary Check

次の日本語に相当する英語を下から選んで記入しなさい。

1. (   )　　顕著な特徴，特質
2. (   )　　きわめて重要な
3. (   )　　有能な
4. (   )　　研究結果，発見
5. (   )　　手に入れる
6. (   )　　機会
7. (   )　　基本的な
8. (   )　　戦略，方策
9. (   )　　傾向，風潮
10. (   )　　適切な，ふさわしい

appropriate／competent／findings／fundamental／hallmark／obtain／
opportunity／strategy／trend／vital

1   Lifelong learning is one of the hallmarks of the nursing profession. While it is a challenge, it is also a commitment that never ends. Nursing's goal is to promote a growing grasp of knowledge and to offer the public the benefit of the very latest innovations. A vital piece of effective
5   health promotion in the public arena is a knowledgeable and competent nurse.

    Continuing education for nurses is usually defined as programs beyond the basic preparation which are designed to promote and enrich knowledge, improve skills, and develop attitudes for the enhancement of
10 nursing practice. It's important to note that not all education takes place in a school setting. Nurses can learn from professional journals that report the latest findings. Many courses are offered in the community by private providers aimed at keeping nurses' knowledge on the cutting edge. Some professional organizations host continuing education classes
15 in conjunction with their meetings. There are also home-study and on-line courses which enhance continuing nursing education. Finally, most

---

Notes

	lifelong learning／生涯学習	*9*	attitude／心構え，態度
	commitment／責任，献身	*9*	enhancement／充実
1	profession／専門職	*10*	practice／業務
2	challenge／挑戦，課題	*10*	note／注意する
3	promote／促進する	*10*	not all ～／すべて～というわけではない
3	grasp／理解，理解力		
3	offer／提供する	*10*	take place／行われる，開催される
3	the public／一般の人々	*11*	setting／環境
4	benefit／恩恵	*11*	professional journal／専門誌
4	latest／最新の	*12*	report／報告する
4	innovation／新しいアイディア，手法	*12*	community／地域社会
5	effective／効果的な	*13*	private provider／民間の提供者
5	health promotion／健康増進	*13*	be aimed at ～／～を目指している
5	public arena／公の場	*13*	on the cutting edge／最先端に
5	knowledgeable／見識のある，聡明な	*14*	organization／団体，組織
7	continuing education／継続教育	*14*	host／主催する
7	be defined as ～／～と定義される	*15*	in conjunction with ～／～と関連して，～と併せて
8	beyond／範囲を超えた		
8	be designed to ～／～するように考えられている	*15*	home-study／自宅学習の
		15	on-line／コンピュータネットワークの
8	enrich／豊かにする	*16*	enhance／高める
9	improve／向上させる		

1   healthcare facilities offer regular in-service courses that assist nurses in obtaining the latest information about healthcare delivery. Simply put, educational opportunities are everywhere.

How do you decide which continuing education programs to attend?

5   A fundamental strategy includes examining your career goals. Where do you want to be in five or ten years? If you like your current job and feel fairly secure, your continuing education courses should be aimed at making you more competent in the things you are doing now. Do not rule out other areas of nursing, though. Technology-based education
10 that teaches you how to surf the Internet, how to e-mail and manage electronic databases, and how to use audiovisual programs will enhance your marketability in the workplace.

An additional strategy for enhancing your flexibility and making you more marketable to future employers includes learning about the areas in
15 which healthcare is moving. So, even if you do not work in managed care or in politics, for example, continuing your education in non-traditional areas can help you in the future. Another example, completing a course in medical Spanish, might make you a more attractive candidate in a multicultural healthcare environment. Likewise, special expertise in

Notes

1	healthcare／保健医療	11	electronic database／電子データベース
1	facility／施設	11	audiovisual／視聴覚の
1	in-service／勤務しながらの	12	marketability／市場性
1	assist A in 〜ing／Aが〜するのを助ける	12	workplace／職場
2	delivery／提供	13	additional／追加の，付加的な
2	simply put／簡潔に言えば	13	flexibility／順応性，柔軟性
4	attend／参加する，出席する	14	marketable／市場性のある
5	include／含む	15	even if 〜／たとえ〜だとしても
6	current／現在の	15	managed care／管理医療
7	fairly／かなり	16	politics／経営，管理
7	secure／安心して，安定している	16	non-traditional／今までになかった，非伝統的な
9	rule out 〜／〜を除外する	17	in the future／今後は，将来は
9	technology-based／科学技術を基盤とした	17	complete／修了する
10	surf the Internet／インターネットからさまざまな情報を得る，ネットサーフィンをする	18	attractive／魅力的な
		18	candidate／候補者
10	manage／管理する，扱う	19	multicultural／多文化の
		19	likewise／同様に
		19	expertise／専門知識

1   bioterrorism might broaden your opportunities to contribute to nursing in other settings.

A popular trend in continuing education for nurses is retraining for different roles. A wide variety of new opportunities are opening up for
5   nurses in community-based roles in home health, managed care, and health promotion, for example. For nurses who have been hospital-based for their entire careers, moving into the community can be overwhelming. Attending an appropriate continuing education course can be a positive way to prepare for this new challenge.

10   The alternative to lifelong learning is stagnation, and no nurse should settle for the status quo. Our patients expect the best; that is what they deserve. And that is what they get from professional nurses who make continuing education an integral part of their nursing careers.

Notes

1	bioterrorism／バイオテロリズム	7	entire／全ての
1	broaden／広げる	7	overwhelming／非常に大変な
1	contribute to ～／～に貢献する	8	positive／積極的な
3	retrain／再教育を受ける	10	alternative／代わりとなるもの
4	role／役割	10	stagnation／停滞
4	a wide variety of ～ ／多種多様な～	11	settle for ～／～を受け入れる，～で
4	open up／広がる		我慢する
5	community-based／地域社会を拠点	11	the status quo／現状
	とする，地域密着型の	12	deserve／値する，受けるに足る
5	home health／在宅医療	13	integral／不可欠な，絶対必要な
6	hospital-based／病院を拠点とする		

練習問題

A　本文の内容に合うように，次の英文の（　　　）内に入る語を下から選びなさい。

① （　　　　　　　　） learning is essential for nurses.

② Examining your career （　　　　　　） is a fundamental strategy when you decide which continuing education programs to attend.

③ Continuing nurses' education in （　　　　　　） areas, such as managed care and politics, might open up new opportunities in the future.

④ A popular trend is retraining for （　　　　　　） roles in home health, managed care, and health promotion.

⑤ No nurse should settle for （　　　　　　）.

community-based／goals／the status quo／lifelong／nontraditional

B　音声を聴いて，次の英文の（　　　）内に適切な語を記入しなさい。

① A triangle can （　　　　　） （　　　　　） （　　　　　） a flat shape with three straight sides and three angles.

② These measures （　　　　　） （　　　　　） （　　　　　） reducing pollution in cities.

③ She （　　　　　） （　　　　　） （　　　　　） （　　　　　） hand-outs.

④ We cannot （　　　　　） （　　　　　） the possibility of lung cancer.

⑤ He （　　　　　） （　　　　　） （　　　　　） public health.

C 次の日本文に合うように，（　　）内の語句を並べかえて英文を作りなさい。

① 両国間の協議はシンガポールで開催されるだろう。
(between, take, Singapore, the two countries, in, the talks, will, place).

② この薬は他の治療法と併用されるかもしれない。
(other treatments, may, with, this medication, conjunction, used, be, in).

③ たとえ走ったとしても，始発の電車には間に合わないだろう。
(catch, run, if, the first train, you, even, won't, you).

D 次の英語に相当する日本語を下から選び，記号で答えなさい【診察】。

① symptom（　　）② blood pressure（BP）（　　）③ pulse（　　）

④ heart rate（HR）（　　）⑤ respiration（　　）⑥ artery（　　）

⑦ vein（　　）⑧ bradycardia（　　）⑨ tachycardia（　　）

⑩ cardiac murmur（　　）

ア．呼吸	イ．動脈	ウ．心雑音	エ．症状	オ．血圧
カ．脈拍	キ．頻脈	ク．静脈	ケ．徐脈	コ．心拍数

Unit 14
The Human Side of Technology

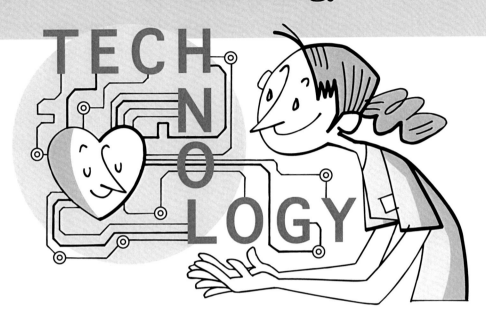

Vocabulary Check

次の日本語に相当する英語を下から選んで記入しなさい。

1. (　　　　　　　　　) 繁栄する，成長する
2. (　　　　　　　　　) ひどく
3. (　　　　　　　　　) 進歩
4. (　　　　　　　　　) 便利なもの
5. (　　　　　　　　　) 厳しい，大変な
6. (　　　　　　　　　) 深刻な，重大な
7. (　　　　　　　　　) 出現
8. (　　　　　　　　　) 物理療法
9. (　　　　　　　　　) 現象，事象
10. (　　　　　　　　　) 唱道する，支持する

advance／advent／advocate／convenience／grave／intense／modality／
phenomenon／severely／thrive

Audio

1   How can anyone be against technology? After all, more people are alive and thriving because of modern technology. We save tiny babies, aged adults, and severely injured persons because of the new technological advances in medical science. How can anyone not value
5   saving lives? However, I must ask this follow-up question: Have *all* of the outcomes from technology been good for nursing and healthcare?

I don't think so. With all of the advances that are supposed to make our lives easier (i.e., faxes, copiers, cellular phones, e-mail, videoconferencing), why aren't our lives any easier? In fact, I would go
10   so far as to say that our lives have become quite a bit more difficult and complex with all of the countless modern conveniences of today. What happened?

Today's modern technology has allowed us to have everything at our fingertips in a matter of seconds. We are saving lives that just a few
15   short years ago would have been lost. And yet, it appears to me that the mood in hospitals has grown more intense and grave than ever before. Why aren't we happier about our new modern conveniences?

In my opinion, with the advent of managed care and the rapid advances of modern technology, we find everyone trying to do more

---

Notes

1	against ～／～に反対して	10	quite a bit／かなり
1	after all ～／だって～だから	11	complex／複雑な
2	because of ～／～のおかげで，～の理由で	13	allow A to ～／Aが～するのを可能にする
4	value／高く評価する，尊重する	13	have ～ at one's fingertips／～をすぐに利用できる
5	follow-up／引き続いての	14	a matter of ～／(時間や距離など)わずかな～
6	outcome／結果，成果	15	and yet／それでも，しかもなお
7	with all ～／～があるものの，～にもかかわらず	15	it appears to A that ～／Aには～と思われる
7	be supposed to ～／～することになっている	16	than ever before／かつてないほどに，従来にも増して
8	i.e.／すなわち(that isに相当するラテン語 id estの略語)	17	be happy about ～／～に満足している
8	copier／コピー機	18	in my opinion／私の考えでは
8	cellular phone／携帯電話	18	managed care／管理医療
9	videoconferencing／テレビ会議	18	rapid／急速な，急激な
9	not ～ any . . .／少しも . . . でない	19	do more with less／より少ない労力と時間でより大きな成果を上げる
9	in fact／それどころか		
9	go so far as to ～／～しさえする		

1   with less. Of particular concern, we find fewer nurses caring for sicker patients. Let me explain.

First, rapid advances in technology make keeping up with new equipment a daily challenge. In past years, we could go to a couple of
5   inservices and one good conference each year and know everything that was important about our specialty area. Today, new equipment and modalities emerge almost *daily*. A huge percentage of our time is spent in keeping up-to-date on new equipment. This is a must; a responsible nurse knows how to use the equipment that is available to benefit all
10   patients.

Second, a fast-growing healthcare phenomenon today is the long-term acute care hospital (LTAC). These hospitals contain patients who were traditionally on the medical-surgical floors of hospitals just a short decade ago. They have been moved here because the medical-surgical
15   floors are now filled with the ICU patients of the 1980s. These patients have been moved from the ICU because the ICU beds are filled with patients who would have been dead 10 years ago without the advances in technology today. Our patients are sicker than they've even been before.

Notes

1	of particular concern／特に懸念されることには	9	benefit／役に立つ，ためになる
1	care for 〜／〜の世話をする	11	long-term acute care hospital (LTAC)／長期急性期ケア病院
3	keep up with 〜／〜に遅れずについていく	13	medical-surgical／内科・外科の
4	equipment／器具，設備	14	decade／10年間
4	a couple of 〜／2，3の〜	15	be filled with 〜／〜でいっぱいである
5	inservice／現職教育コース	15	the ICU patients of the 1980s／1980年代なら集中治療室（intensive care unit）にいたであろう患者
8	up-to-date／最新の情報に通じて		
8	must／絶対に必要なこと		
9	available／利用できる，入手可能な		

1   Finally, much like our counterparts in the corporate world, we are doing more with less. Nurses are the largest personnel pool in any healthcare institution, so when economic indicators demand cuts, the first place the ax usually falls is in the nursing pool.

5   In summary, I propose that the new era of technology has certainly benefited nurses and the way we do our jobs. However, we must continue to adamantly advocate safe patient care within this new era, as we attempt to do more with less. We must use technology and all of its advances to help us do our jobs more effectively.

Notes

1	counterpart／よく似た人	5	in summary／要するに
1	corporate／企業の	5	era／時代
2	pool／集まり，一団	7	adamantly／断固として
3	economic indicator／経済指標	8	attempt to ～／～しようと試みる
4	ax／斧	9	effectively／効果的に

練習問題

A 次の英文が，本文の内容と一致する場合にはTを，一致しない場合にはF
を（　　　）内に記入しなさい。

（　　　）① The author believes that modern technology is not useful for
nursing and healthcare.

（　　　）② Our lives would be more difficult and complicated without today's
modern technology.

（　　　）③ Only a limited nurse is demanded to keep up with the latest
equipment.

（　　　）④ The ICU beds are full of patients who would have been dead 10
years ago without the advances in technology..

（　　　）⑤ It is nurses that will be fired first when a hospital is in financial
difficulties.

B 音声を聴いて，次の英文の（　　　）内に適切な語を記入しなさい。

① I wouldn't （　　　　　）（　　　　　　　）（　　　　　　　）（　　　　　　　）
（　　　　　　　） say that she's a liar.

② I was able to identify the thief （　　　　　）（　　　　　　　）（　　　　　　　）
（　　　　　　　） seconds.

③ （　　　　　）（　　　　　　　）（　　　　　　　）, it's the best car on the market.

④ The cafeteria （　　　　　）（　　　　　　　）（　　　　　　　） students during
lunch time.

⑤ The patient （　　　　　）（　　　　　　　） rise but fell down.

C 次の日本文に合うように，（　　）内の語句を並べかえて英文を作りなさい。

① そのお金のおかげで私は留学できた。
（study, the money, to, me, allowed, abroad）.

② 私にはあなたは思い違いをしているように思われる。
（mistaken, me, appears, you're, it, that, to）.

③ 私たちの生活は以前よりずっとストレスが多くなっている。
（before, than, our lives, stressful, more, get, ever）.

D 次の英語に相当する日本語を下から選び，記号で答えなさい【治療や療法】。

① inhalation（　　）② suction（　　）③ dialysis（　　）

④ enema（　　）⑤ blood transfusion（　　）⑥ intubation（　　）

⑦ chemotherapy（　　）⑧ organ transplantation（　　）

⑨ suture（　　）⑩ incision（　　）

> ア．切開　イ．挿管　ウ．吸引　エ．縫合　オ．輸血
> カ．臓器移植　キ．吸入　ク．化学療法　ケ．浣腸　コ．透析

Unit 15

A Vision for Nursing

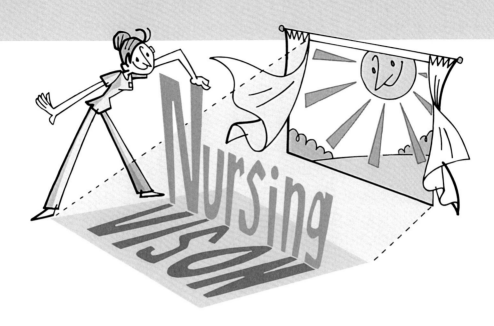

Vocabulary Check

次の日本語に相当する英語を下から選んで記入しなさい。

1	(	)	最先端，最前線
2	(	)	利権
3	(	)	最善の，最適の
4	(	)	利用，活用
5	(	)	再入院
6	(	)	慢性の
7	(	)	回復する
8	(	)	小児科の
9	(	)	老年の，高齢者の
10	(	)	更年期，閉経期

chronic／forefront／geriatric／interest／menopause／optimal／pediatric／
rehospitalization／restore／utilization

1　　How has professional nursing evolved to its present state? Do you wonder if there was a great master plan? Are we exactly where great thinkers thought we would be 30 years ago? Or, have we just happened?

5　　If we want to make nursing better in the future, we must take control; we must have a vision of nursing in the year 2040 and create a viable plan for reaching that vision.

　　I believe our vision must be one that focuses on nurses at the forefront of health—health delivery, health promotion, health maintenance, and
10　health restoration. I see nurses as the leaders of healthcare, the access and departure point for every health need for every patient. Much like physicians were in the 1980s before managed care fragmented access and care, I think nurses should be the gatekeepers of healthcare.

　　We must have a vision where ancillary groups, such as physicians,
15　healthcare institutions, private insurers, and special interest groups, support the work that nursing does to keep people physically and mentally healthy. Nurses have to focus on our public health, mental health, and health promotion prowess to become the nation's primary healthcare provider of choice.

1   No one should enter or leave the gated community of health delivery without a nurse who is responsible for their primary healthcare before, during, and after their encounter. This responsibility should be in collaboration with the patient. Nurses should approach each member of

5   the public in a partnership role for optimal utilization of health services. We can certainly call on our ancillary services if our patients need brain surgery, gait training, or in-hospital care for a few days. However, the promotion, management, and restoration of their health should be a nursing responsibility, guided and controlled by one nurse.

10   We must have a vision in which nurses partner with insurers and government entities to provide health services in a more cost-effective way. The savings related to reducing and managing pain, decreasing rehospitalization, reducing recurring chronic problems, improving the quality and quantity of life, and restoring dignity to the dying process

15   are all nursing-based savings opportunities.

Nurses being seen as the nation's primary healthcare provider of choice, the gatekeepers of healthcare—now that is a vision.

Nurses partnering with government and private insurers to provide health promotion, maintenance, and restoration—that is a plan.

Notes

1	gated community／門のある社会（本来は，治安のためフェンスなどで囲み，警備員が門で出入りをチェックする住宅地のこと）	6	brain surgery／脳外科手術
		7	gait training／歩行訓練
		7	in-hospital／入院中の
2	be responsible for ～／～に対して責任がある	10	partner with ～／～と組む
3	encounter／出会い	11	government entity／政府機関
3	responsibility／責任	11	cost-effective／費用対効果の高い
3	in collaboration with ～／～と協力して	12	saving／救助，救済
		13	recurring／繰り返し発生する
5	partnership／協力，提携	14	dignity／尊厳
6	call on ～／～に要求する，～に頼む		

1   Once we have established this shared vision for nursing, ideas and strategies will begin to take shape. Pediatric nurse practitioners will find solutions to the problem of uninsured children. Geriatric nurse practitioners will take charge of the nursing home industry and fix it.

5   Women's health will focus on the natural aspects of menstruation, childbirth, and menopause instead of making them medical problems. Complementary therapies will decrease the over-dependence on pharmaceutical agents currently experienced by so many elders. *Health* care will replace *illness* care.

10   Once the benefits of being educationally prepared for a clear role as the gatekeepers of healthcare have been clearly articulated, undereducated nurses will reenter the nursing education system and prepare for their future roles. This infusion of new students will increase nursing educator needs, resulting in higher salaries and inducing younger nurses to choose

15 education as a career option. And, if the current educational systems do not meet the needs of the emerging workforce, they will be replaced with newer on-line, user-friendly educational approaches for preparing nurses for the vision of our future.

    The future of nursing is ours. If we grasp it, we will thrive. If we

Notes

1	once 〜／いったん〜すると	8	elder／年長者
1	shared／共通の	9	replace／とって代わる
2	strategy／戦略，方策	11	articulate／明確に表現する
2	take shape／具体化する，実現する	11	undereducated／教育不足の
2	nurse practitioner／ナースプラクティショナー	12	reenter／再び入る
3	uninsured／無保険の	13	infusion／注入
4	take charge of 〜／〜を受け持つ，〜を預かる	14	result in 〜／〜という結果に終わる
4	nursing home／老人ホーム	14	induce A to 〜／Aに勧めて〜させる
4	fix／回復させる，正常な状態に戻す	16	meet／満たす
5	menstruation／月経	16	emerging／新興の，発展中の
6	instead of 〜／〜の代わりに，〜ではなくて	16	workforce／労働力
7	complementary therapy／代替療法	16	be replaced with 〜／〜に取って代わられる
7	over-dependence／過度の依存	17	on-line／コンピュータネットワークの
8	pharmaceutical agent／医薬品	17	user-friendly／使いやすい
		19	grasp／つかむ
		19	thrive／成長する，繁栄する

1　timidly decline to get involved, we will be left behind. Someone else will rise to claim healthcare and move it in their direction. If we miss this opportunity to be the shapers of the future of healthcare, the quality of patient care and the nursing profession itself will suffer.

5　　What is your vision for nursing? I challenge you to move forward and make professional nursing better than it is now. The future of nursing is too important to be left to chance.

Notes

1	timidly／臆病に	4	profession／専門職
1	decline to ～／～することを断る	4	suffer／苦しむ，損害を被る
1	get involved／関わる	5	challenge A to ～／Aに～するようにあえて要求する
1	leave ～ behind／～を置き去りにする	7	too ～ to ...／～すぎて…できない
2	claim／自分のものだと言う	7	leave ～ to chance／～を成り行きに任せる
2	miss／逃す，逸する		
3	shaper／形づくる人		

練習問題

A 次の英文が，本文の内容と一致する場合にはTを，一致しない場合にはF
を（　　）内に記入しなさい。

（　　）① The author argues that nurses should be the leaders of
healthcare.

（　　）② Physicians used to be the gatekeepers of healthcare.

（　　）③ Geriatric nurse practitioners will fix the problem of uninsured
elderly people.

（　　）④ If younger nurses choose to reenter the nursing education
system, there might be a chance for them to get promoted.

（　　）⑤ If nurses miss the opportunity to be the shapers of the future of
healthcare, the quality of patient care will be worse.

B 音声を聴いて，次の英文の（　　）内に適切な語を記入しなさい。

① The study will be performed （　　　　　　）（　　　　　　）（　　　　　　）
the government.

② I will （　　　　　）（　　　　　　）（　　　　　　） this new class.

③ The traffic accident （　　　　　）（　　　　　　） the death of two
drivers.

④ Old cups （　　　　　） gradually （　　　　　）（　　　　　） new ones.

⑤ Don't （　　　　　） your health （　　　　　）（　　　　　）.

C 次の日本文に合うように，（　　）内の語句を並べかえて英文を作りなさい。

1 いったん彼女が仕事を見つけると，事態は好転した。
(a job, better, things, found, got, she, once).

_____

2 彼女は勉強しないで午後ずっとテレビを見ていた。
(all afternoon, studying, watching TV, of, she's, instead, been).

_____

3 私は彼に決心するようにあえて要求した。
(his mind, him, up, to, challenged, make, I).

_____

D 次の英語に相当する日本語を下から選び，記号で答えなさい【検査】。

1 physical examination（　　） 2 urinalysis（UA）（　　）

3 endoscopy（　　） 4 complete blood count（CBC）（　　）

5 angiography（　　）

6 electrocardiogram（ECG，EKG）（　　）

7 catheter（　　） 8 contrast medium（　　） 9 gastroscopy（　　）

10 biopsy（　　）

ア．造影剤　イ．血管造影　ウ．生検　エ．カテーテル　オ．心電図
カ．身体検査　キ．胃カメラ検査　ク．尿検査　ケ．全血球計算
コ．内視鏡検査

Stories for Nurses － 英語コラムで読む看護師の物 語

2022 年 12 月 10 日　第 1 版　第 1 刷 ⓒ
2024 年 3 月 20 日　第 1 版　第 2 刷

編　著　　田中　芳文
発 行 者　　濱崎　浩一
発 行 所　　株式会社看護の科学新社
https://www.kangonokagaku.co.jp

東京都新宿区上落合 2-17-4　〒 161-0034
☎ 03（6908）9005
印刷・製本／スキルプリネット
DTP／スタジオ・コア

Printed in Japan

ISBN978-4-910759-11-1